The Thyroid Alternative

*Renew Your
Thyroid Naturally*

Dr. Nikolas R. Hedberg

D1565856

The Thyroid Alternative

By Nikolas R. Hedberg, D.C., D.A.B.C.I.

Published by:
Renew Your Health, LLC
141 Asheland Ave. Suite 301
Asheville, NC 28801

Dr. Hedberg's Office:
828-254-4024
www.drhedberg.com

Printed in the United States of America
First Edition

ISBN-13: 978-0-6154-2823-9
ISBN-10: 0-615428-23-1
Paperback $19.95

Book Designed by Steven Peterson
Edited by Gloria Shen

Warning-Disclaimer:
Renew Your Health, LLC has designed this book to provide information in regard to the subject matter covered. It is sold with the understanding that the publisher and the author are not liable for the misconception of misuse of the information provided. Every effort has been made to make this book as complete and as accurate as possible. The purpose of this book is to educate. The author and Renew Your Health, LLC shall have neither liability nor responsibility to any person or entity with respect to any loss, damage, or injury caused or alleged to be caused directly or indirectly by the information contained in this book. The information presented herein is in no way intended as a substitute for medical counseling.

This book is dedicated to all of my patients with thyroid problems. I have learned so much from you and I am honored that you trust me with your health care. I am truly grateful for the opportunity you have given me to serve you.

Forward

Dr. Nikolas Hedberg, a gifted functional medicine physician and respected colleague, has done a masterful job at explaining the extremely complex subject of endocrinology from a functional perspective in this book. Thyroid disorders are occurring at epidemic proportions in the Western world, particularly the U.S., and there are many reasons for this. Dr. Hedberg tackles many of these difficult issues, including the role of stress, lifestyle, diet, toxins, and autoimmunity in thyroid disease. If you are suffering from a thyroid problem this book is a must read. It will allow you to understand all the complex factors that may be playing a role in your condition, and it will prepare you to serve as a knowledgeable self-advocate with your physicians, who often do not recognize, nor appreciate, all of these associated factors. It will allow you to exhaust all possible options in addressing your condition, while improving your overall health in the process, before resorting to hormone replacement therapy. If hormone replacement therapy is required you will understand all of your options, and not just the ones generally presented to you by standard primary care physicians and endocrinologists who do not practice from a functional medicine perspective.

Sincerely,

David M. Brady, ND, DC, CCN, DACBN
Vice Provost, Health Sciences Division
Director, Human Nutrition Institute
Associate Professor of Clinical Sciences
University of Bridgeport (Bridgeport, CT)
Private Practice: Whole Body Medicine (Trumbull, CT)

Contents

Introduction

It is estimated that 70-90 percent of deaths in the U.S. are not genetic but are modifiable through diet, exercise and the reduction of environmental toxin exposure. This stands in the face of traditional medical education which teaches treatment of disease through drugs and surgery rather than a comprehensive individualized analysis of each individual's unique case. Traditional physicians are not trained or qualified to implement nutrition, diet, exercise and other lifestyle changes to patients' treatment plans leaving little hope for healing chronic disease. Doctors are taught about drugs by agents of the pharmaceutical industry who work hard to persuade these physicians to select the newest and most expensive medications even in the absence of scientific evidence that these drugs are any better than older, less costly ones. This situation exists despite the fact that there is plenty of evidence to support that non-drug interventions are more effective and less costly.

Between 1990 and 2000, health care costs increased by 69 percent per capita in the US to $4,637.[1] Germany ranked number two in the world and yet US per capita costs were 68.5 percent higher than Germany and 2.5 times greater than costs in the UK.[2] Prescription drugs were responsible for 21 percent of this increase.[3] In 2001, our total spending was $1.4 trillion.[4] By 2011, spending is expected to rise to $3.1 trillion.[5] This model is becoming more and more costly as the numbers of sick individuals steadily increase requiring more resources for care. Our health care system does very well with emergency medicine for things such as accidents, traumas, rampant infections and life-saving surgeries. However, with chronic disease, it fails miserably. The biggest threats to our health are social isolation, obesity, increasing stress, lack of exercise, undernutrition from hollow food, and industrial pollution of our air, water and earth.

The United States is currently ranked 37th in overall health care among industrialized nations despite the fact that we spend more money per person than any other country. One of the main reasons our health care system is so poor is due to the fatally flawed model that encourages waiting until symptoms and disease arise before action is taken. Prevention is not a priority in our health care model. Even so called preventative procedures such as mammograms fail to deliver much usefulness in preventing breast cancer. The reason that our health care system is structured the way it is can be explained by the strong pharmaceutical influence on medical education, training and practice. Drugs do not prevent disease; they merely mask symptoms and do not correct the underlying causes of a disease. This model neatly categorizes a set of symptoms that have a named disease and then a drug that is designed to "treat" this disease is prescribed. Whatever the drug may be, it does not address the underlying physiological imbalances that resulted in disease in the first place. Hypothyroidism is a perfect example of how this model does not deliver. Patient A goes to her doctor and is diagnosed with hypothyroidism. A synthetic form of thyroid hormone is then prescribed to alter the blood test to a "normal range" and hopefully improve symptoms. This is a great model for the drug companies and the prescribing doctor but not for patients. This model does not ask the question: "Why is the thyroid out of balance?"

Patients are then dependent on their doctor and the drug company to continually monitor and adjust their medication for life. As you can see, this is a highly profitable model for the doctor and for the drug company.

What if the underlying cause of the thyroid imbalance were uncovered, corrected, and the patient were educated on how to keep her thyroid in balance? This would remove the dependence on the doctor and drug company resulting in major financial losses to both parties. Many patients are scared into taking medications by their doctors; we have been conditioned to think that medical doctors know all and know what's best for us. In the public eye, MDs can be trusted to have our best interest at heart. That is, of course, true for some but even those doctors are practicing a model that does not correct underlying physiological imbalances that lead to disease. Thomas Edison is famous for saying, "The doctor of the future will give no medicine, but will interest his patients in the care of the human frame, in diet and in the cause and prevention of disease." This eloquent statement is coming true as more and more alternative medicine doctors are practicing and even traditional MDs are learning a new model of health care.

Approximately one in ten Americans suffer from hypothyroidism and as many as ten percent of women have inadequate thyroid hormone production. The most common cause of hypothyroidism is Hashimoto's autoimmune thyroid which causes chronic inflammation and slow destruction of the thyroid gland. Hashimoto's is an autoimmune condition meaning that the body is producing antibodies that attack your own tissue which in this case is the thyroid gland. You may have a thyroid problem if you have any of the following symptoms:

- **Fatigue**
- **Sluggishness**
- **Increased sensitivity to cold**
- **Constipation**
- **Pale, dry skin**
- **A puffy face**
- **Hoarse voice**
- **An elevated blood cholesterol level**
- **Unexplained weight gain**
- **Muscle aches, tenderness and stiffness**
- **Pain, stiffness or swelling in your joints**
- **Muscle weakness**
- **Heavier than normal menstrual periods**
- **Brittle fingernails and hair**
- **Depression**

After reading many existing books on the thyroid, I decided that it was time to educate everyone on the underlying causes of thyroid dysfunction and the necessary steps required to heal the thyroid and optimize its functioning. This book is designed to give you, the reader, an understanding of how the thyroid works, what causes it to become dysfunctional, and how to find out what's causing the dysfunction. There is a great deal of information published on the thyroid and how to treat it with conventional or alternative medicine but nothing on finding the underlying cause of the imbalances. In order to understand how the thyroid should be evaluated and treated, you must understand a functional model versus a replacement model of treatment. Traditional Western medicine is the best example of how a replacement model of treatment works. Let's say you go to your traditional doctor complaining of some thyroid symptoms such as fatigue, depression, constipation and extreme cold sensitivity. Your doctor may run a blood test to evaluate the thyroid and if the results show hypothyroidism, you are given a drug that was designed to address your symptoms and the lab test. This model is fatally flawed because it doesn't ask the question as to why the thyroid is not functioning properly. This is true for many other conditions in Western medicine where drugs are given to treat lab tests and symptoms without a thorough evaluation of why the body is out of balance in the first place.

A functional model will also run blood tests but also other lab tests to find out why the thyroid is out of balance. Once the imbalances are identified via laboratory testing, natural medicines, nutrition, detoxification and lifestyle modifications are used to correct the imbalances. The functional model does not require patients to be dependent on their doctor as opposed to a Western replacement model which requires them to keep going back to fill their prescription. A functional model finds the imbalance and corrects it. Your doctor will also teach you why the imbalance happened in the first place and how to prevent it from coming back. You may need some repeat testing to monitor treatment and make changes in supplementation, diet and lifestyle until you are well. This is what true healing is, not taking toxic medications that only suppress symptoms, have side effects that can be devastating, and do not correct the underlying cause of why you were sick in the first place. Natural medicines that are used in a functional model rarely have side effects and are not required for long periods of time.

The thyroid is a perfect example of how a Western replacement model fails so many people because there are a multitude of other factors that can affect thyroid function. These include the following which we will get into more detail in each chapter:

- **Lyme Disease**
- **Rickettsial infections**
- **Epstein-Barr Virus**
- **Intestinal dysbiosis (abnormal gut bacteria)**
- **Adrenal gland dysfunction**
- **Blood sugar imbalances**
- **Impaired liver detoxification**
- **Essential fatty acid status**
- **Heavy metal toxicity**
- **Thyroid-disrupting chemical exposure**
- **Vitamin & mineral deficiencies**
- **Gluten intolerance**
- **Insulin resistance**
- **Autoimmune Disease**
- **Excess estrogen**
- **GI infections**
- **Mitochondrial dysfunction**

Did your doctor do the necessary detective work and evaluate these potential causes of your thyroid problem? Or were you just given a medication and told you would have to take if forever? I see this all too often in my practice. Patients are not thoroughly evaluated and do not get well on medication.

Many alternative practitioners are guilty of using a replacement model as well. Patients are given natural supplements that are made for the thyroid gland, but again the underlying causes of the imbalances are not uncovered and corrected. This is no doubt a safer approach than medication but it establishes the same dependency on the doctor except the patient needs to keep coming back for more supplements instead of medication.

This book is written for you, the patient who wants a thorough understanding of how the thyroid becomes dysfunctional and how you should be evaluated by a functional medicine practitioner. You will also learn that your symptoms may actually have nothing to do with your thyroid and could be from other imbalances in your body. It is very important to understand that everything in your body is connected meaning that when your health is compromised, there can be many underlying imbalances that must be corrected in order for you to get well.

CHAPTER ONE
The Thyroid

The thyroid is a small gland that lies in the neck about the level of the Adam's apple and weighs approximately one ounce. It produces thyroid hormone and calcitonin. The parathyroid glands are very small and lie on the outside portion of the thyroid gland and secrete parathyroid hormone. We will be focusing on thyroid hormone.

The thyroid gland is stimulated to make thyroid hormone by thyroid-stimulating hormone (TSH) which is produced in the pituitary gland located in the brain. The pituitary is controlled by the hypothalamus in the brain which monitors the amount of circulating thyroid hormone. Iodine must enter the thyroid gland through a transport system that is repaired with the intake of vitamin C. There is usually about 20-30 mg of iodine in the body and 75 percent of it is stored in the thyroid. In addition to iodine, magnesium, zinc, copper, and vitamins B2, B3, and B6 are required for thyroid hormone production.

The thyroid gland produces two thyroid hormones: T4 (thyroxine) and T3 (triiodothyronine). Ninety-five percent of thyroid hormone produced is T4 and five percent is T3. T3 is the active form of thyroid hormone which is produced as a result of one iodine being cleaved from T4. T4 is inactive so the majority of thyroid hormone produced is actually inactive. The numbers "3" and "4" indicate the number of iodines. This is key in understanding optimal thyroid function. Both T4 and T3 are bound to proteins in the blood until they reach your cells and become unbound to work their magic on metabolism.

Most of the T4 is converted into T3 in the liver. Approximately sixty percent of the T4 is converted into T3, twenty percent is converted into an inactive form of thyroid hormone known as reverse T3 (irreversible), and the remaining twenty percent is converted into T3S (T3 sulfate) and T3AC (triiodothyroacetic acid).

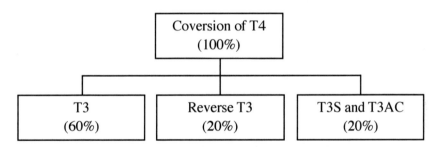

Figure 1: Conversion of T4 in the Liver

Reverse T3 can be problematic; even though it is inactive, it will still bind to T3 receptors and block T3 from binding and working its magic on metabolism. Too much or too little cortisol that is produced by the adrenal glands will increase circulating levels of reverse T3. This mechanism is due to suppressed liver detoxification and clearance of reverse T3 from excess cortisol production. Stress can not only cause signs of hypothyroidism but it will also impair the liver's ability to detoxify. Cortisol will also suppress TSH production resulting in low thyroid function. Immune system activation, high adrenaline, excess free radicals, aging, fasting, stress, prolonged illness, and diabetes will also drive the inactivation of T3 to reverse T3.

Problematic Aspects of Reverse T3

Has the ability to bind to T3 receptors which will block T3 from binding and working its magic on metabolism.

Is impacted by several factors in an individual's system:
- Too much or too little cortisol will increase circulating levels of T3
- Selenium deficiency
- Immune system activation
- High adrenaline
- Excess free radicals
- Aging
- Fasting
- Stress
- Prolonged illness
- Diabetes will also drive the inactivation of T3 to reverse T3

T3 and reverse T3 can also be inactivated by conversion into a hormone known as T2. Elevated insulin levels due to a diet high in refined carbohydrates will also increase reverse T3 levels. Toxic metals including mercury, cadmium and lead will also increase reverse T3 production. T3S and T3AC are inactive until they are catalyzed by an enzyme in the GI tract known as sulfatase. This enzyme is dependent on healthy gut bacteria. We will discuss in a later chapter the importance of a healthy digestive tract as it relates to twenty percent of active thyroid hormone.

Thyroid hormone's main role is to control metabolism (energy production) inside the cell. Our cells contain tiny factories called mitochondria that produce energy from fat, sugar and protein. Thyroid hormone controls the function of the mitochondria which determines how much energy is produced. Symptoms of low thyroid function are related to a decrease in energy production including:

- **Fatigue**
- **Weight gain/inability to lose weight**
- **Constipation**
- **Dry/itchy skin**
- **Dry brittle hair and nails**
- **Depression**
- **Headaches**
- **Overly sensitive to cold**
- **Cold/numb hands and feet**
- **Muscle cramps**
- **Depressed immune system–can't recover from infections**
- **Slow wound healing**
- **Unrefreshing sleep**
- **Digestive problems due to low stomach acid**
- **Hair falls out**
- **Water retention**
- **Lateral third of eyebrow thinning**

TSH

Traditional medicine relies mainly on the TSH or thyroid-stimulating hormone blood test to measure thyroid function. TSH is not a thyroid hormone. TSH is produced by the pituitary based on how much thyroid hormone is circulating in the bloodstream. As thyroid hormone levels drop, TSH production will increase to stimulate the thyroid to make more hormone. If thyroid hormone increases, then TSH production will decrease because the thyroid is making plenty of hormone. The TSH alone is not adequate to assess thyroid function because it doesn't take into consideration the conversion of thyroid hormone into its active form which occurs in the liver, kidneys and lungs. The TSH test also does not take into account thyroid hormone receptor resistance. Thyroid hormone receptors can become resistant to thyroid hormone due to thyroid-disrupting chemical exposure leading to normal blood tests but development of low thyroid symptoms. Cortisol produced during stress by the adrenal gland can also inhibit TSH production further throwing off the accuracy of the test. If the TSH is elevated, the traditional physician will prescribe synthetic T4 and this will usually reduce TSH into the "normal" range. This approach does not take into account peripheral thyroid hormone conversion or receptor binding. If the body is compromised in its ability to activate thyroid hormone into T3, then taking T4 will result in a failure of treatment. If the adrenal glands are out of balance, then most likely thyroid hormone function will also be out of balance. In addition, if thyroid hormone receptors are desensitized, this approach will fail as well.

You will find that most medical physicians do not spend much time reading the peer-reviewed medical literature which provides us with valuable data on TSH levels. An excellent study was published by Obal and Krueger (2001) on sleep deprivation and thyroid hormone production. The researchers concluded: "When sleep deprivation is maintained for weeks, the plasma concentrations of T4 and particularly T3 decline but TSH remains normal."[6] Do physicians ask you about your sleep patterns? Perhaps this could be the reason for the abnormal TSH. I have seen many patients who also suffer from insomnia and sleep problems and present with low thyroid symptoms and abnormal TSH levels. Does this mean they should have thyroid hormone dumped into their bodies? Unfortunately, this happens to many people. I always take into account every patient's sleep pattern and correct it as part of our treatment plan. Many times, sleep patterns are abnormal due to blood sugar and adrenal gland imbalances. Remember, you are not a lab test but a beautiful, complex being where everything is connected as one.

Testing & Diagnosis

Blood tests alone cannot always adequately diagnose thyroid hormone imbalance. It is estimated that about forty percent of the U.S. population suffers from some kind of thyroid imbalance as opposed to the current traditional figure of ten percent. This is due to the inadequacies of the TSH test. In addition to blood testing, I review a thorough case history and a number of detailed health questionnaires and also perform a comprehensive physical examination for clues to thyroid hormone imbalance. Basal body temperature testing is used by many practitioners to evaluate thyroid function but this does not solely indicate a thyroid imbalance. There are many other factors that can cause a low basal body temperature such as adrenal fatigue, leaky gut, impaired liver detoxification and malnutrition. I use the basal body temperature simply as one more diagnostic tool to evaluate the overall picture of a patient. Another sign that may indicate low thyroid function is thinning of the lateral one-third of the eyebrow.

The following thyroid tests can provide more information about your thyroid. Use this as a guide when you get the results of your blood tests:

TSH (Thyrotropin) – Thyroid-stimulating hormone is produced by the pituitary to stimulate the thyroid to make hormone. The ideal range is 1.8-3.0. Traditional medicine uses a much broader range of 0.5-5.5. This range misses many hypothyroid patients such as those with a TSH between 3.0-5.5.

Total Thyroxine (T4) – This test measures the amount of T4 (thyroxine) that is both bound to protein and unbound.

Free Thyroxine Index – This is calculated by multiplying the TT4 by the T3 uptake. The result gives you the amount of unbound T4 or Free T4.

Free Thyroxine (Free T4) – This measures the amount of unbound or free T4 which is the most active form. Free T4 is not affected by medications or other factors that affect protein bound thyroxine (TT4).

T3 Uptake – A measurement of the amount of available binding sites for free T3 on thyroxine-binding proteins. Elevated testosterone will reduce the number of binding sites and cause a low T4 and high T3 uptake. Excess estrogen from hormone replacement or birth control pills will increase binding sites and can cause high T4 and low T3 uptake.

Free Triiodothyronine (Free T3) – This is a measure of free T3 levels or unbound T3. This is the best test if your natural physician wants to see the amount of available active thyroid hormone in the bloodstream.

Reverse T3 (rT3) – This is a measurement of the amount of T3 that has been inactivated.

Thyroid Antibodies – Thyroid peroxidase, thyroid-stimulating immunoglobulin and antithyroglobulin elevations indicate autoimmune thyroid disease such as Hashimoto's or Graves' disease. Thyroglobulin and calcitonin are mainly used in the diagnosis of more serious thyroid diseases such as cancer.

Prescription Medications

Prescription medications do not take into account underlying physiological imbalances and may lead to dependence on the medication. The following drugs are prescribed by physicians to treat the thyroid:

Synthroid – Synthetic thyroxine (T4). Synthroid is the most popular prescription drug for hypothyroidism. Synthroid is in the top five most commonly prescribed drugs in the US. Synthroid can be converted incorrectly into inactive reverse T3 resulting in no symptom improvement. Synthroid depletes calcium for bones and may not provide improvement for patients who have compromised conversion pathways of T4 into T3 or any of the other imbalances described in this book.

Levoxyl – Synthetic thyroxine (T4).

Levothroid – Synthetic thyroxine (T4).

Levothyroxine – Synthetic thyroxine (T4).

Thyrolar – Synthetic T4 and T3.

Cytomel – Synthetic T3. Many side effects including hyperthyroid symptoms.

Armour Thyroid, Nature Thyroid, Westhroid – Natural thyroid hormone from desiccated pig thyroid tissue. Contains approximately 38 micrograms/grain of T4 and 9 micrograms of T3/grain as well as other cofactors for thyroid hormone production. Nature Thyroid is a better choice than Armour because it does not contain corn and other binders.

Many alternative-minded medical doctors prescribe Armour and other natural dessicated pig thyroid tissue. This is a better option in some cases than merely prescribing synthetic T4 (Synthroid) because these natural agents also contain T3. The problem with Armour is that it contains corn and other fillers which can be a problem for those with specific sensitivities. Nature Thyroid is the best choice because it doesn't contain corn or fillers. But the author does not agree with this treatment method because even though it is a better option, it still does not take into account the underlying causes of why the thyroid is out of balance in the first place. These natural prescriptions still only replace thyroid hormone and require dependence on the doctor for continued prescriptions and office visits. I have seen many, many patients who are on such natural prescriptions who still have many symptoms and have been taking the prescription for a long period of time. Even if someone responds to a prescription such as Armour thyroid, she should be rigorously evaluated for underlying physiological imbalances.

Another issue with such treatment methods is suppression of hypothalamic-pituitary-thyroid feedback mechanisms. Whenever you take a hormone that is produced in the body, this tells the brain that it no longer needs to stimulate hormone production because it is constantly being ingested. When male bodybuilders take testosterone, their testicles shrink because there is no longer a need for them to make testosterone. Taking thyroid hormone for long periods of time will suppress natural production which may or may not return after discontinuing the medication. It is strongly encouraged that you do everything possible to normalize thyroid function before going on medication of any kind. Americans typically want a quick fix, a magic pill that will instantly give relief. Many people get this instant relief from medication but the long-term effects of dependency and suppression of natural hormone production may not be worth it. Patients who have had their thyroid removed or partially removed may require prescription thyroid hormone. If the gland is not present then thyroid hormone must be replaced. In this case, prescriptions such as Armour and Nature Thyroid are the better choice.

Conversion of T4 into T3

T3 is much more active than T4 and is responsible for most of the actions of thyroid hormone on the cell. Some people cannot convert T4 into T3 as efficiently as others. In addition, there are many factors that could be inhibiting this process.

Selenium, antioxidants, iron, magnesium, zinc, vitamin A, vitamin B6 and B12 deficiencies can lead to poor conversion. The medications listed above affect thyroid hormone conversion as well as production and receptor binding. As people get older, they lose their ability to convert thyroid hormone which may be due to decreased vitamin and mineral absorption. This is due to a loss of intestinal barrier function where all of your nutrition is absorbed. This barrier loses its function as we age so supplementation is absolutely necessary. Excess estrogen from xenoestrogens in the environment, birth control pills and hormone replacement can lead to low thyroid symptoms. Estrogen increases the protein that binds to thyroid hormone leaving excess thyroid hormone bound to protein which is inactive until it becomes unbound. Cortisol produced by the adrenal gland is a major factor in converting thyroid hormone. Too much cortisol can inhibit the activation of thyroid hormone and too little cortisol yields the same result. Exhausted adrenals will cause low thyroid symptoms due to the lack of cortisol production. Insulin is a hormone released by the pancreas to handle blood sugar elevations after consumption of carbohydrates and can inhibit hormone conversion as well. Soy products have been shown to inhibit the conversion of thyroid hormone. This only goes for soy products that are non-fermented. Fermented soy products such as miso and tempeh are okay.

Vitamin C has been shown to enhance the conversion of thyroid hormone. Radiation, chemotherapy, growth hormone deficiency, and cigarette smoke have also been shown to reduce thyroid hormone conversion. We will get into more detail of how these imbalances can affect thyroid hormone function and production in each chapter.

CHAPTER TWO
Autoimmune Thyroid

The number one cause of hypothyroidism in the world is Hashimoto's autoimmune thyroiditis. Autoimmune thyroiditis is also the most common undiagnosed autoimmune disease in the world. More women are diagnosed with this condition than men. Many patients do not receive a thorough evaluation of their thyroid gland and are put on thyroid medication without adequate testing for autoimmune thyroid. Patients with autoimmune thyroid usually do not respond to medication and their doctors are continually adjusting their medication based on lab tests. The TSH test can significantly fluctuate in autoimmune thyroid due to the immune system's attack causing inflammation of the thyroid. Traditional medicine does not check for autoimmune thyroid routinely which leaves patients with true autoimmune thyroid in limbo for months and even years before their doctor finally decides to run tests for autoimmunity. Even in these cases it is sad because the treatment for autoimmune thyroid is medication. That's right, the treatment is the same for you whether you have autoimmune thyroid or thyroid dysfunction that is not autoimmune.

There is definitely a familial factor in autoimmune thyroiditis but not necessarily a genetic factor. Habits of living tend to run in families such as food choices, lifestyle, acid-forming diets, and eating patterns that promote poor digestion, all of which can contribute to the development of autoimmune disease.

In autoimmune thyroiditis, thyroid cells are attacked by the body's own immune system causing destruction of the thyroid gland and chronic inflammation. It can cause an overactive thyroid or underactive thyroid – the latter being the most common. Most frequently, the thyroid is slowly attacked over time leading to hypothyroidism with an elevated TSH (thyroid-stimulating hormone). Traditional medicine treats Hashimoto's with synthetic T4 (thyroxine) and when the TSH is in the normal range, the patient is considered to be treated successfully. The autoimmune component is rarely addressed which does the patient a great disservice because the body's attack can be greatly reduced sparing the thyroid gland for a much longer period than without treatment. Many of these patients continue to take synthetic thyroid hormone but still have symptoms of hypothyroidism.

Graves' disease is another form of autoimmune thyroiditis which is characterized by hyperthyroid activity with symptoms of anxiety, insomnia, eye-bulging, weight loss, swelling in the thyroid gland, and either increased or decreased energy depending on what stage. Graves' is more prevalent in women with an 8:1 ratio of female to male. It usually occurs between the ages of twenty and forty. Hyperthyroid symptoms include anxiety, nervousness, sweating, weight loss, fatigue and insomnia. The thyroid is producing too much thyroid hormone in these cases which will result in signs of increased metabolism in the beginning; however, over time as thyroid receptors become saturated and the gland begins to lose function, signs of hypothyroidism begin to emerge. The underlying cause of Graves' and Hashimoto's can be the same so we still approach these cases not from a disease model but from a cause-effect model. What triggered the autoimmunity in the first place?

Graves' disease is treated with medications that shut down thyroid function including methimazole, propylthiouracil and radioactive iodine obliteration. Instead of trying to heal the thyroid gland, some traditional physicians will destroy the thyroid gland with radioactive iodine. Once this is done, the patient must remain on thyroid hormone forever. I have saved many thyroids from radioactive iodine treatment and the patients have not required thyroid hormone replacement to function optimally.

Carnitine and Graves' Disease (Hyperthyroidism)

L-carnitine is a di-peptide that shuttles fat into the cell's mitochondria (mini energy-producing factories) so it can be burned to make energy. A paper was published in 2004 in the Annals of the New York Academy of Sciences in which the authors found:

L-carnitine is a peripheral antagonist of thyroid hormone action. In particular, L-carnitine inhibits both T3 and T4 entry into cell nuclei. This is relevant because thyroid hormone action is mainly mediated by specific nuclear receptors. In the randomized trial, we showed that 2 and 4 grams per day of oral L-carnitine are capable of reversing hyperthyroid symptoms. L-carnitine was acting in the periphery, namely as an inhibitor of thyroid hormone action in thyroid hormone target tissues, and not at the level of the thyroid gland as an inhibitor of thyroid hormone synthesis. Overall the two doses of carnitine (2 and 4 grams) were equally effective in reversing hyperthyroid symptomatology; asthenia, nervousness, and palpitations were the symptoms that benefited the most. Amelioration occurred 1 or 2 weeks after commencement of carnitine.[7]

So as you can see, L-carnitine is a must for all Graves' disease patients. I use a liquid form that delivers high doses and is cost-effective as L-carnitine tends to cost more than most supplements.

Autoimmune thyroiditis tends to be an innocent bystander with other autoimmune diseases such as Type 1 diabetes, rheumatoid arthritis, lupus, etc. Most doctors chase these other autoimmune diseases ignoring the possibility that the thyroid is also being attacked.

Patients with autoimmune thyroiditis tend to have symptoms that lead them to explore abusive and addictive behaviors to help deal with the devastating effects of this condition. Depression, anxiety, hopelessness, extreme fatigue and weight gain can be very difficult to deal with. Alcohol is one outlet for such people as it is readily available and provides instant results when one is feeling down. The problem is of course an increasing need to drink regularly to deal with like symptoms. These people truly need help and can be led to full recovery. These are also the patients who are sent to a psychiatrist for medication specific to their symptoms. They end up on thyroid hormone and then antidepressants or anxiety meds which further impair thyroid and immune system function. How I wish I could get these patients to see me before they become entangled in the toxic traditional medical system.

Autoimmune thyroiditis can begin when the thyroid gland becomes more permeable meaning that there is increased blood flow into the gland as well as substances that should not enter the thyroid. This is a sign that the blood-thyroid barrier has been breached and white blood cells enter the gland and attack it. This also indicates that the body can no longer keep up and repair the damage that is done by the immune system. This can many times be traced to an intestine that is hyperpermeable allowing unwanted substances and toxins into the blood further exhausting the body's repair reserves. As the gut becomes more permeable or "leaky," so do the rest of the body tissues including organs such as the thyroid, brain, kidneys etc. It's important to understand that autoimmune thyroiditis is not a singular disease process but a symptom of a broken down immune system due to a variety of possible causes which we will cover in detail.

We have already covered the symptoms of hypothyroidism which include mainly fatigue, difficulty losing weight, temperature dysregulation, loss of memory and hardship getting started in the morning. When you wake up, it is the T4 (thyroxine) and T3 produced by the thyroid gland that increase your temperature. If there is an autoimmune attack on the thyroid, this will impair its ability to make the relevant hormone which leads to low body temperature and difficulty getting going in the morning. Remember that stress hormones can inhibit thyroid hormone receptors so even if there is normal thyroid hormone production, you may still have all the symptoms of hypothyroidism. This is why the adrenal glands are so important in all types of thyroid dysfunction. Thyroid hormone receptors can become dysfunctional due to not only stress hormones but also metabolic acidosis, environmental toxins, toxic heavy metals or antibodies that specifically attack the receptors. This further emphasizes the importance of a thorough investigation into the causes of your symptoms and not just a TSH blood test.

Many patients with autoimmune thyroiditis seek care for other problems in the beginning of their disease process. Some of these include increased allergies, asthma, irritable bowel syndrome, sleep problems and weight gain. They go to specialists such as allergists, gastroenterologists, sleep clinics, etc. but end up without help. This is due to the fact that specialists only look at these diseases and symptoms from their myopic view of health and disease. If only the body were not compartmentalized by these physicians but looked at as one entity that is fully connected in every way with every part of itself, people would have answers to their health problems.

A skilled physician will be able to feel your thyroid gland to see if it is enlarged or if there are nodules. I have encountered some traditional physicians who do not think it's possible to feel nodules on the thyroid. After telling them to perform an ultrasound to confirm my findings, there have always been nodules on the thyroid that I have felt. The swelling occurs due to increased water in the thyroid due to the inflammation caused by the immune attack on the thyroid. Usually the thyroid gland is the most swollen in the beginning stages of disease and then slowly shrinks in the advanced stages due to an inability to compensate. Can the thyroid gland regain its original size and function? The answer is yes as long as everything is done right to remove all underlying causes of autoimmunity and to provide the thyroid with the proper nutrition that it needs.

As a natural physician, it is my goal to find the underlying causes of disease and correct the imbalances. It is important to understand that once the gene is expressed causing autoimmune disease, it will never turn off. At least at this point, no one knows how to manipulate our genes in such a way. What we can do is balance the immune system which greatly reduces the immune attack on the thyroid cells. We will now discuss the many faces of autoimmune thyroid.

Candida

Candida and other yeasts can contribute to the development and perpetuation of autoimmune thyroiditis. Yeasts that grow in the intestine suppress immune function and acidify the digestive environment. Yeasts also impair absorption of important nutrients that are required for immune function. In some cases the yeast is so bad it regurgitates into the stomach causing chronic heartburn and impaired digestion. Yeasts can also hold onto toxic chemicals and metals which are released when commencing an anti-yeast program. This is one of the reasons why some people get sick when following such regimens. Patients with yeast overgrowth also have impaired intestinal barrier function allowing these toxins to freely enter the bloodstream further taxing the immune system. Yeast overgrowth is a sign of poor diet, impaired immune function and a diet that is too acidic. In some cases, the yeast must be slowly killed as the immune system is supported simultaneously. Multiple probiotic strains of at least forty billion viable organisms must be consumed each day during this process. If the immune system is still weak, the diet is poor, and supplements are not taken, then the yeast can quickly grow back. Constipation can further worsen this problem as yeasts feed on sugars that are produced from food that is fermenting in the intestine due to a prolonged transit time. Food should pass through the entire digestive system in twelve to eighteen hours so it does not have time to ferment. Increasing transit time is a first order of priority when eradicating yeast overgrowth. A stool analysis will provide data on the type of yeast and what natural compounds will kill the yeast. This test is very important as some yeasts are completely resilient to natural medicines that are known to kill yeast. The lab report contains what is known as a "sensitivity" meaning the yeast has been exposed to multiple natural agents looking for what works and what doesn't. For example, the lab may report that garlic does not work for a particular yeast but oil of oregano does work.

Molecular Mimicry

Molecular mimicry is an important aspect to understand as a possible cause of Hashimoto's disease. The body's immune system works by recognizing amino acid sequences which make up protein but the foreign invader looks the same as self tissue. Amino acids are the building blocks of protein and make up body tissues, foreign invaders and of course dietary proteins such as gluten and casein from milk. Molecular mimicry occurs when a dietary protein or infection contains protein that the body's immune system attacks but is identified as the same protein found in body tissue such as thyroid cells. According to Tomer et al. in the journal Endocrine Review (1993), "Molecular mimicry has long been implicated as a mechanism by which microbes can induce autoimmunity."[8]

Yersinia enterocolitica is a bacterium we can get from contaminated food and water and is one example of an infectious agent that can trigger autoimmune thyroid. The protein that makes up the outer shell of Yersinia can lead to cross-reactivity or molecular mimicry of thyroid tissue resulting in an immune attack on Yersinia and the thyroid gland. Yersinia has actually been found to have TSH binding sites on its surface. As long as the Yersinia infection resides in the intestine, the body will continue to produce antibodies that attack the bacteria and the thyroid. Eradication of the infection will eliminate or significantly reduce the autoimmune attack on the thyroid gland. I have found that most of my patients with autoimmune thyroiditis have a chronic infection that is driving the autoimmunity. Lyme disease and it's associated co-infections (Babesia, ehrlichia, bartonella, mycoplamsa etc.) tend to be the most common infections that trigger autoimmunity.
Examples of infections that can induce autoimmune thyroid include:
Epstein-Barr Virus- causes mononucleosis or "mono."
Lyme disease spirochete (Borrelia burgdorferi)- *bacteria transmitted by biting insects.*
Rickettsia- *bacteria transmitted by biting insects.*
Hepatitis C – *virus that resides in the liver.*

Herpes virus – *incurable virus found in the nervous system.*
Parvovirus B19 – *virus that causes "fifths disease" in children and can affect adults.*
Influenza B – *The classic "flu" virus.*
Rubella – *virus that causes German measles.*

Insulin Resistance and PCOS
Insulin resistance that leads to polycystic ovarian syndrome (PCOS) can lead to autoimmune thyroid. PCOS is not only the most common cause of infertility in the US but also the most common female hormone disorder. PCOS is identified by increased cholesterol, triglycerides and blood sugar in routine blood testing. In addition, an elevated testosterone hormone test is diagnostic for PCOS. As the name suggests, PCOS can present with one or many ovarian cysts. Chronic surges of blood sugar causing insulin surges lead to increased androgen production in the ovaries leading to PCOS. Insulin receptors no longer respond to insulin causing the pancreas to release excess levels of insulin further feeding the vicious cycle. Elevated testosterone and insulin have been shown to result in autoimmune thyroid. Your natural physician will have a protocol for insulin resistance which has been extremely successful in a short period of time in my practice.

Vitamin D
Adequate vitamin D levels can be achieved only by sunlight exposure or supplementation. Vitamin D has been found to be associated with autoimmune thyroid. Vitamin D helps to balance the immune system that is out of balance and attacking the thyroid gland. Patients with autoimmune thyroid disease have been shown to be deficient in vitamin D with genetic abnormalities in their vitamin D receptors. Even normal levels of vitamin D in these individuals

will not be enough leading to requirements of much higher doses of supplementation. Lack of sunlight, gastrointestinal inflammation, aging, darker skin and elevated cortisol can cause a vitamin D deficiency. All autoimmune thyroid patients must be tested for vitamin D deficiency but the traditional laboratory reference ranges are not optimal and miss many deficiencies. Your natural physician will know how to interpret these tests and guide you with proper supplementation. 2,000 IU is the absolute minimum daily dose for vitamin D supplementation. Autoimmune patients need between 2,000-10,000IU/day especially if their receptors are genetically abnormal requiring higher doses.

Gluten

It has been proposed that the immune system tags certain foods such as gluten but also TSH receptors on the thyroid gland resulting in attack on not only the food but the thyroid gland as well. Gluten is a protein found in many grains including wheat, barley, rye, oats, and spelt. Celiac disease is a disease that first appeared approximately 10,000 years ago during the development of agriculture in the Fertile Crescent. The first symptoms that were documented were chronic diarrhea, abdominal distension and muscle wasting. It was not until 1950 that a young Dutch pediatrician named Dicke made the association between gluten and disease. He was the first to implement the gluten-free diet as a cure for celiac disease. It was then in the 1960s that the genetics of gluten intolerance began to emerge in research.

Celiac patients have approximately ten times the rate of autoimmune thyroid diseases such as Hashimoto's and Graves' disease as non-celiac individuals. It has been shown in the literature that 26.2 percent of celiac patients have autoimmune thyroid disease.[9] Celiac disease and gluten intolerance are not the same condition. Celiac disease is the devastating autoimmune condition that significantly breaks down the intestinal barrier causing immune dysfunction, malabsorption of nutrients and many problems outside of the intestine. In fact, 70 percent of gluten's effects can be outside of the intestine including multiple organ system disorder which results in dysfunction of organs such as the thyroid, liver, adrenals, pancreas, sex organs, heart, brain, bones, and kidneys.

Gluten intolerance may not have an autoimmune component so the effects are not as devastating as celiac disease. Gluten intolerance can still result in damage to the intestine and extra-intestinal organ dysfunction but is usually not as severe. Many people live their entire lives with gluten intolerance but never even know it. They may suffer from mild to moderate health problems such as osteoporosis, nutritional deficiencies, hypothyroidism, digestive problems and even autoimmune thyroid. The degree of gluten intolerance depends on genetics, environment, nutrition and, of course, how much gluten is consumed.

Gluten is hidden in many packaged foods and commercial products. Gluten intolerance has an extremely strong link to autoimmune thyroid disease. The body will produce antibodies to gluten but they will cross-react and also attack the thyroid gland. This is called molecular mimicry. Many people are gluten-intolerant and are not aware of it. It is a mistake to think that if you don't have any digestive problems, you don't have a gluten issue. Remember, 70 percent of gluten's negative effects occur outside of the intestine affecting other tissues including the thyroid gland.

Patients who have celiac disease or gluten intolerance must avoid gluten indefinitely. A strict gluten-free diet must be followed in these cases. Gluten-free guidelines are presented in the thyroid diet chapter.

Vitamin B12

Hashimoto's patients have been shown to be deficient in vitamin

B12 which causes a condition known as pernicious anemia. Vitamin B12 requires a substance called intrinsic factor to be absorbed but sometimes the body produces antibodies to intrinsic factor resulting in a lack of B12 absorption. Many times, gluten intolerance and B12 deficiency go together because gluten sensitivity affects the three main factors in vitamin B12 absorption:

1. Adequate hydrochloric acid production in the stomach.
2. Pancreatic enzymes.
3. A healthy small intestinal lining.

Your doctor will order intrinsic factor antibodies if you are unresponsive to vitamin B12 supplementation. Sublingual B12 bypasses the gut and is an excellent delivery system to raise B12 levels. B12 injections provide the most efficacious route of administration.

Iodine

As discussed in a previous chapter, iodine is a very important nutrient for the health of the thyroid gland. Too much iodine or iodine consumption in autoimmune thyroid can exacerbate the immune attack on the thyroid gland. The enzyme in the thyroid that is under attack is stimulated by iodine thus leading to an increased attack on the gland. It has been shown that iodine supplementation in an autoimmune thyroid patient leads to increases in the thyroid peroxidase antibody. It has also been found that when iodine is added to table salt in iodine-deficient areas, the rate of autoimmune thyroid illness increases. There is a tremendous amount of controversy at this point on the use of iodine for thyroid function and other parts of the body. Until there is more definitive research available, iodine is not recommended in most cases for autoimmune thyroiditis at this point due to the potential of worsening the condition.

Mercury

A 2006 study found that removal of mercury-containing dental amalgam resulted in decreased levels of thyroid antibodies thus reducing the intensity of the attack on thyroid cells.[10] Patients with autoimmune thyroid were tested for mercury sensitivity and those that were positive had their dental amalgams removed resulting in decreased antibody levels after six months.

Mercury is one example of how an environmental toxin can trigger autoimmune disease. Toxins disrupt normal immune function and can alter tissue proteins making them look foreign to the immune system cells. Continuous exposure to a toxin such as mercury can lead to immune system dysfunction, culminating in autoimmune disease. Mercury is one of the best examples because it binds to proteins and enzymes altering their structure which confuses the immune system.

These toxins get into the system by passing through the barrier systems of the body. These include the intestinal barrier, lung barrier, skin barrier and blood-brain barrier. Leaky gut is a major problem in our society due to high stress (cortisol eats away at the intestinal barrier), poor diets, toxins, infections and gluten sensitivity. Leaky gut can increase the chances of autoimmune disease.

If the blood-brain barrier is leaky, toxins such as mercury can pass into the brain and cause immune cell dysfunction in the neurons of the brain. Treating the barrier systems of the body with natural medicine is an integral part of overcoming the negative effects of autoimmune disease. It is important to understand that we are all exposed to environmental toxins on a daily basis but our overall health and genetics determine how we handle and detoxify them. Some individuals can live a long healthy life despite constant exposure and some will suffer from severe debilitating sickness with even the smallest exposure.

The Barrier Systems

Understanding the barrier systems is vital to understanding the onset of autoimmune disease in some cases. The barrier systems are composed of four parts:

1. Intestinal barrier
2. Lung barrier
3. Skin barrier
4. Blood-brain barrier

The gut has mucosal barriers that prevent the entry of foreign invaders into the body. They are called the barrier system because they are the first line of defense from the outside world. When the gut barrier breaks down, the result is a localized or systemic inflammatory cascade by the immune system. "Leaky gut" or gut hyperpermeability describes this condition and it is not only related to autoimmune thyroiditis but also psoriasis, autoimmune diseases, allergies, asthma, malabsorption, inflammatory bowel and skin problems such as eczema and dermatitis. There are a few laboratory tests that will diagnose this condition and all are readily available. The first is the lactulose/mannitol test. The patient drinks a solution of the two sugars, lactulose and mannitol, and then urine is collected for six hours. Lactulose is a very large sugar and if it ends up in the urine in sufficient quantities, this indicates leaky gut. Mannitol is a small sugar and should pass through easily but if it doesn't, this indicates malabsorption. You can have a leaky gut and also malabsorption. The second test is the intestinal barrier function blood test. This is a direct measure of aerobic and anaerobic bacteria, dietary proteins and yeast activity in the intestinal barrier. If these markers are sufficiently elevated, then we can say the intestinal barrier is broken. The third test is an indirect measure of the gut barrier known as food sensitivity testing which we will discuss in more detail.

Aristo Vojdani, Ph.D. has said, "When the barriers are broken, the results will be autoimmunity." Stress (high cortisol), infections (bacteria, parasites, viruses, yeast, fungi), drugs, antibiotics, NSAIDS (non-steroidal anti-inflammatories such as aspirin, ibuprofen, etc.), steroids, antacids, antibiotics, alcohol, allergens, constipation, immune system imbalances, xenobiotics, dietary proteins such as gluten, enzymes, constipation due to inadequate fiber intake, poor digestion and environmental toxins can all break down the intestinal barrier which is 70 percent of your body's immune system. NSAIDS cause bleeding and inflammation in the GI tract resulting in significant mucosal barrier damage. Antacids impair normal stomach acid function causing compromised protein digestion. This leads to large undigested proteins entering the small intestine which are then absorbed into the bloodstream taxing the immune system. Low stomach acid also causes mineral deficiencies in calcium and magnesium. Antibiotics disrupt normal flora not only in the intestinal tract but also the skin, vagina, and mouth, potentially leading to yeast infections in these areas. The yeast that overgrows in the intestine can result in bloating, gas, chronic fatigue, depression and gut inflammation.

The following nutrients can become depleted due to leaky gut: vitamins A, C, E, B-complex, zinc, selenium, CoQ10, magnesium calcium, essential fatty acids, choline, inositol, glutathione and sulfur amino acids. Disorders such as cirrhosis of the liver, hepatitis, irritable and inflammatory bowel, ulcers, colon cancer, low stomach acid and diverticulosis/itis can all lead to gut hyperpermeability as well. The cells that line the intestine have the highest turnover rate and thus are the most vulnerable to nutrient deficiencies. These cells mainly feed on the amino acid glutamine, which when supplemented, has been shown to reverse leaky gut.

When the gut bacteria become out of balance, the intestinal barrier is adversely affected. This can occur from antibiotic use which eliminates not only good but bad bacteria and can result in yeast overgrowth as well. Replenishing "good" bacteria such as lactobacillus and bifidobacter can reverse this imbalance and help heal the intestinal barrier. Prebiotics known as fructooligosaccharides (FOS) provide food for beneficial strains of bacteria. Diets high in simple sugars and excess meat can lead to constipation thus increasing the amount of time that the gut barrier is exposed to toxins.

Chronic inadequate stomach acid production can lead to depressed intestinal immune function and can result in small intestinal bacterial overgrowth. As the intestinal barrier breaks down, food allergies begin to increase, the immune system begins to function abnormally and the result can be autoimmunity. The intestinal barrier is composed of tight gap junctions that allow nutrients from the food we eat to pass into the bloodstream. When the intestinal barrier breaks down, a condition known as "leaky gut" or "hyperintestinal permeability" can occur. This means that undigested food particles and foreign invaders can pass into the system without resistance. This constant overload of foreign invaders is a continuous stress on the immune system that over time will lead to immune system dysfunction. Your immune system knows exactly what is going on in every part of your body but it can only do so much. If it constantly has to "clean up" what shouldn't be there, it may eventually break down from overwhelming stress.

The lung barrier is constantly exposed to air pollution, secondhand smoke and off-gassing of toxic chemicals from products such as new automobiles (that new car smell is not good!), carpeting, dry-cleaned clothes, paint, solvents, furniture, wrinkle-free clothes, new plastics, and many building materials. These will stress the lung barrier and break it down leading to increased toxin exposure into the blood.

The skin barrier's main enemy is excessive washing practices by those in industrialized nations. Bathing and washing excessively can break down the skin barrier leading to increased absorption of environmental toxins. Many of the commercial products available today are loaded with chemicals that break down the skin barrier and contain thyroid-disrupting chemicals. Cosmetics, soaps, body wash, shampoos, conditioners, lotions, after-shave, etc. are extremely toxic and a broken skin barrier will only allow increased absorption of these chemicals into the bloodstream.

There are two very important things to consider when discussing what products to use. The first is that if something is on your skin, you are basically drinking it. Your skin will absorb almost everything you put onto it. The second thing to consider is that you shouldn't put anything on your skin unless you would eat it. Use only all-natural products made from plants that won't harm your skin or your insides.

The blood-brain barrier begins to break down after the intestinal barrier has begun to break down. The blood-brain barrier is extremely selective in what it allows to pass in and out of the brain. This should be quite obvious as brain tissue is very delicate. As the blood-brain barrier breaks down, substances that wouldn't normally pass into the brain end up passing through causing an immune response and inflammation in the brain. The immune cells of the body begin to attack what has crossed the blood-brain barrier but unfortunately, they don't always attack the foreign substance and harm normal brain tissue as well.

So as you can see, the barrier systems are very important in maintaining a healthy immune system and preventing autoimmunity. Addressing the barrier systems is a key factor in overcoming autoimmune disease including autoimmune thyroid. The main target is the intestinal barrier which can be measured through a blood test called the "intestinal barrier function" test. This test tells your natural physician the integrity of the intestinal barrier and can gauge treatment time and level of aggressiveness.

The first aspect that needs to be addressed when healing the intestinal barrier is to eliminate any infections that may reside in the intestine. This can be a parasite, bacterium, virus or yeast overgrowth such as candida. It is also important to take beneficial bacteria to replenish the healthy colonies that may have been disrupted from the infection. And finally, supplements that have been shown to rebuild the intestinal barrier should be taken through this process. Daily physical exercise that is not too strenuous is important in healing the gut. Massage and therapeutic biofeedback are passive modalities that can help to reduce stress. A high-fiber diet to ensure proper transit time of food through the gut as well organic, whole, unprocessed foods are mandatory for healing. Identify and avoid toxic exposures from chemicals, metals and allergens to facilitate healing. It will be very difficult to heal the gut as long as there is intake of NSAIDS, antacids, steroids or antibiotics. Essential nutrients such as fatty acids, vitamins, minerals, and amino acids in fully bioavailable form should be supplemented.

One of the main causes of intestinal barrier breakdown is stress. Counseling and group therapy can greatly aid in stress reduction. You must perform regular stress-reduction techniques such as meditation, yoga, tai chi, prayer, exercise.

Food Sensitivities

The next most important thing in repairing the intestinal barrier and improving immune function is to avoid food sensitivities. Each time you eat a food to which your body's immune system reacts, it further breaks down the intestinal barrier and taxes the immune system. This can increase the autoimmune attack on the thyroid gland. There are a few different ways to find out if you are sensitive to a particular food. The first is to have a blood test that measures a large number of different foods and the level of reaction your body is having to each one. This is a fast and easy way to pinpoint what foods you should avoid while your intestinal barrier is healing. This is an excellent measure of the integrity of the intestinal barrier and immune function. The second way is to go on an elimination diet which is done by avoiding the most common food allergens which include: dairy, gluten, soy, tomato, peanuts, corn and eggs. This is done for three to six months while the intestinal barrier is healing. The purpose of this diet is to remove immune stresses on the intestine so it can heal. Each time you eat a food that your immune system is sensitive to, it stresses the intestinal barrier further breaking it down. Testing usually consists of a blood sample taken and analyzed for a large number of food reactions. Each food is graded on a scale indicating a mild, moderate or strong response. The more food sensitivities that show up as well as the number of moderate-to-strong responses can indicate the integrity of the intestinal barrier. As the foods are eliminated and the barrier heals, the immune system will no longer react to these foods as before. Some foods need to be avoided indefinitely or on rotation even when the barrier is healed to prevent a relapse.

Alcohol, NSAIDS (non-steroidal anti-inflammatories) and aspirin should be avoided as they contribute to the breakdown of the intestinal barrier. Constipation must also be eliminated which can be done with increased fiber intake, drinking half your bodyweight in ounces of water each day, doing a "vitamin C flush", and taking probiotics (acidophilus, bifidobacter etc.), FOS, and magnesium. If this doesn't resolve the constipation, then there are other underlying causes that need to be evaluated. Seven to nine hours of sleep each night should be a top priority when healing the gut lining. This is when the majority of healing takes place, so do whatever you can to get adequate sleep. Coffee, tea and soda must be eliminated or extremely restricted during this process as well. The following supplements have been shown to repair and aid the intestinal barrier in healing: L-glutamine, Zinc-carnosine, Vitamin A, Aloe Vera, MSM, Folate, DGL (licorice), Slippery Elm, Marshmallow Root, Quercetin, Prunus, N-Acetyl Glucosamine, Cat's Claw, Okra, Mucin, and Chamomile.

Diagnosis & Treatment

Many patients with symptoms of thyroid dysfunction are not properly tested for the causes of imbalance. There are two antibodies that should be tested by blood: thyroid peroxidase and antithyroglobulin antibodies. These antibodies are elevated in 85-90 percent of chronic thyroiditis patients. Thyroid peroxidase is the enzyme required for thyroid hormone synthesis and if these antibodies are positive, it indicates the body's immune system is attacking this enzyme. Thyroglobulin is a protein found in the thyroid gland and if these antibodies are positive, it indicates that the immune system is attacking this particular protein in the thyroid gland. In either case, if one or both are elevated, then the diagnosis of autoimmune thyroiditis can be made. In addition, ANA (antinuclear antibody) can be elevated in cases of Graves' disease.

Thyroid nodules can occur in autoimmune thyroiditis due to inflammation and damaged thyroid tissue cells. Nodules can appear in four to seven percent of the US population but have also been found in up to fifty percent of the population upon autopsy. Thyroid nodules can be felt by a skilled physician. If a nodule is found on physical examination, an ultrasound should be performed to provide more detailed diagnostic information. Thyroid cancer can result from autoimmune thyroiditis and should be ruled out.

Chapter Conclusion

Many people ask the question if the thyroid can regain normal function once there is autoimmunity. The answer is yes in a vast majority of cases. If the attack on the thyroid has been too intense and prolonged, then the thyroid cells may simply be dead and cannot regenerate. If however, the imbalances are found before this happens, the thyroid may achieve full recovery. As with all patients, it is my main goal to find the underlying physiological imbalance through laboratory testing, correct the imbalances through nutrition, lifestyle and proper supplementation, and to teach each patient how to maintain a high level of health removing dependency on myself or any other physician.

CHAPTER THREE
The Gut-Thyroid Connection

Many diseases can be traced to a breakdown in the gastrointestinal tract where 70 percent of your immune system resides. The GI tract has many important functions for overall health including digestion, nutrient absorption, elimination, detoxification, hormone metabolism and energy production. Every brain chemical known as a neurotransmitter is also found in the intestine where 99 percent of neurotransmitters are made. The GI tract is very important when achieving optimal thyroid health.

Remember that T4 (thyroxine) is inactive until it is converted into T3 (triiodothyronine) which is the active form of thyroid hormone. Twenty percent of the thyroid hormone in your body must be converted into the active form (T3) in the GI tract by the enzyme sulfatase. This is a significant percentage considering the powerful role that thyroid hormone plays in the body. This conversion of inactive thyroid hormone into active thyroid hormone in the GI tract is dependent on healthy colonies of beneficial bacteria. An imbalance in the ratios of bacteria in the GI tract (dysbiosis) can lead to low thyroid function. This explains why so many patients with thyroid hormone imbalance also have digestive problems and normal thyroid blood chemistry panels.

In addition, there is another mechanism in the GI tract that can lead to low thyroid function. Your digestive tract is lined with lymph (immune) tissue known as GALT (gut-associated lymphoid tissue). Stress to the GALT from food sensitivities, undigested proteins, leaky gut, and infections from bacteria, yeast and parasites can cause a major stress response which raises cortisol production by the adrenal glands. Cortisol will cause a shift in thyroid hormone metabolism increasing the inactive form of T3 known as reverse T3. Approximately twenty percent of thyroid hormone is converted into the inactive reverse T3 but this percentage will be even higher if there is an offending agent in the GI tract.

Chronic elevations in cortisol from stress will suppress the immune system in the GI tract which will lead to dysbiosis, parasites, yeast and leaky gut which then creates a vicious cycle further disrupting thyroid function. As you can see, the GI tract is extremely important in optimizing thyroid function. I have seen many patients whose thyroid function normalized after simply treating imbalances in the GI tract.

Excess estrogen in the body can suppress thyroid hormone function by binding to thyroid hormone receptor sites. The GI-Estrogen-Thyroid relationship is very important in optimizing thyroid function. The GI tract contains an enzyme called beta glucuronidase that can reactivate estrogen that has been metabolized in the liver. The metabolized form of estrogen would normally be excreted in the feces but in the face of too much beta glucuronidase, it can be reabsorbed into the bloodstream. This enzyme is dependent on optimal nutrition and healthy gut bacteria ratios. Once again we see how important healthy gut bacteria are to the health of the thyroid. Poor diet, stress, toxins, unresolved psychological issues, inadequate stomach acid production and digestive enzymes can lead to dysbiosis (abnormal bacterial ratios).

GI-Liver-Thyroid Connection

Hormones and toxins are metabolized in the liver and excreted in the feces through the GI tract. Remember that a majority of thyroid hormone is converted into its active form in the liver. When the GI tract is out of balance from dysbiosis, inflammation, leaky gut, infections or too many food allergies, this puts a major strain on the liver's ability to metabolize hormones and thyroid-disrupting chemicals. This leads to a toxic liver impairing its ability to activate thyroid hormone. This scenario also increases the chances of thyroid-disrupting chemicals recirculating and impairing thyroid function. This continues the vicious cycle of the enzyme beta glucuronidase which undoes what the liver has done to metabolized hormones which may be reactivated and reabsorbed into the bloodstream and the liver.

When the intestinal barrier is broken, autoimmune thyroid may result. Infections such as candida, parasites and bacteria are a constant stress on the adrenal glands and also contribute to chronic inflammation. These infections must be eliminated in order to have optimal thyroid function. Your natural physician will order a stool analysis to diagnose GI infections. These tests will also tell you how well you are digesting and absorbing food, if there is inflammation and if you have sufficient beneficial bacteria to convert some of your thyroid hormone into its active form.

Determining if You Have a Digestive Problem

If you are having digestive problems, there is a good chance that it is affecting your thyroid function. Bloating after meals, gas, cramping, loose stools, constipation, burping, heartburn, and inconsistent stool formation can all be signs of a digestive problem. You can begin to see if you have digestive problems by doing an easy test at home. This is known as the transit time test.

Food should pass through your intestines in 18-24 hours. If it takes longer than twenty-four hours, there is something wrong with your digestive tract. This easy to do test can be done at home to measure food transit time.

Purchase a product called "activated charcoal" which is an inert substance and will turn your stool black or dark gray.

Swallow four capsules with a meal and write down the day and time that you take the capsules.

Observe your stool until you see black or dark gray stool appear. At this point, write down the day and the time. Look at the time that you originally swallowed the capsules and the time that you see the dark stool and write down the total time it took for this to happen. If it took longer than twenty-four hours, you have some work to do on your digestive tract. If it took less than 18 hours, that may also be a problem meaning that there is something irritating the digestive tract causing increased peristalsis.

The best way to determine if you have problems in your digestive tract is to complete a stool analysis. This will be ordered by your functional medicine physician. I recommend testing through Metametrix laboratory. They offer a profile called a GiFX Comprehensive Stool Analysis. Metametrix uses cutting edge technology for microbe detection in stool. This test will tell you if you have any infections that could be affecting the thyroid gland. It also tells you how well you are digesting food, if you are absorbing the food you are eating, if you have any yeast overgrowth, parasites, fungus, and/or mold and whether you have an inflammatory bowel versus an irritable bowel. It even tests for gluten intolerance. This test will also reveal if you have intestinal dysbiosis which is basically an imbalance in the bacterial colonies in the gut. This test is vital for everyone who has autoimmune thyroiditis because of the possible infectious triggers in the gut.

How to Address Imbalances in a Stool Analysis
If there are any imbalances found in the stool analysis, the following guidelines should be followed:

Perform the "4 R's" of gastrointestinal dysfunction:
Remove: Eliminate known food allergens such as gluten, dairy, eggs, soy, peanuts, etc. Blood testing can pinpoint food reactions. Alcohol, caffeine and NSAIDS should be avoided as well. A stool analysis will diagnose infections that can be eliminated with natural medicines or medications.

Repair: Supplements to repair the intestinal barrier are taken.

Replace: Hydrochloric acid and pancreatic enzymes offer digestive support.

Reinoculate: Probiotics that contain friendly bacteria such as lactobacillus and bifidobacter are taken to reinoculate proper bacterial colonies.

CHAPTER FOUR
The Liver & Detoxification

The liver is an extremely complex organ involved in multiple immune and metabolic processes. If the liver is not detoxifying optimally, it will be virtually impossible to have success with any disease including thyroid and hormone imbalances. Unfortunately, many patients are given hormones without a thorough analysis of their liver's ability to metabolize hormones. This can do more harm than good due to a build-up of unmetabolized hormones or incompletely metabolized hormones circulating in the blood- stream causing abnormal hormone responses. Partially metabolized hormones can bind to hormone receptor sites blocking normal hormones from binding and causing abnormal responses.

Nutrition, toxin exposure and genetics are all key factors in liver detoxification. I have seen many patients who were put on hormones and had impaired liver detoxification systems only to result in a worsening of their condition and even cancer from excess estrogen. Many studies have shown that impaired liver detoxification can lead to fatigue and autoimmune disease – both major factors in thyroid health. The majority of thyroid hormone is converted into its active form in the liver. If the liver is not functioning optimally, signs and symptoms of hypothyroidism will arise. The liver is also important for balancing sex and adrenal hormones due to its role in metabolizing hormones and detoxifying thyroid-disrupting chemicals. The process of detoxification is basically the conversion of fat-soluble compounds into water-soluble compounds that can be eliminated in the feces, urine and sweat. Hormones are fat-soluble compounds as well as environmental toxins, drugs, pesticides, and allergy-causing complexes.

There are two distinct phases of liver detoxification known as Phase I and Phase II. Phase I involves the cytochrome P450 enzymes and Phase II involves six pathways: glucuronidation, acetylation, sulfation, methylation, glycine conjugation, and glutathione conjugation. Liver enzymes can directly neutralize chemicals or convert them into waste products that can be easily excreted by the body.

Inflammation can put undue stress on the liver but can be reduced by compounds such as zinc, curcumin, fish oil and alpha-lipoic acid. L-carnitine, l-methionine, choline and inositol all help to metabolize fat in the liver-enhancing function and can reverse fatty liver disease. Phosphatidylcholine (from lecithin) can protect from liver alcoholic cirrhosis.

Insulin resistance puts major stress on the liver due to inefficient sugar-burning in the liver which leads to fatty acid production from the excess sugar. Over time, this leads to fatty liver disease.

A leaky gut will put undue stress on the liver due to a constant flow of toxins passing through the gut barrier and entering the liver which must then detoxify these compounds.

The following pathways must be supported for proper detoxification. This can be important for thyroid patients who have thyroid imbalances due to excess testosterone, estrogen, toxic metals and thyroid disrupting chemicals.

Sulfation Support

Sulfation basically involves binding toxins with sulfur-containing amino acids so they can be excreted. The enzyme used in this step is dependent on molybdenum. Sulfur-containing amino acids include methionine, glycine and n-acetyl-cysteine.

Glucuronidation Support

Glucuronidation occurs when toxins are bound to glucuronic acid which is produced by the liver. B-vitamins, glycine and magnesium are required for this process.

Methylation Support

Methylation is required for compounds that have been altered in Phase I detoxification. This process requires folate, SAMe, methylcobalamin (B12), magnesium, trimethylglycine, pyridoxal-5-phosphate(B6), choline, vitamin E, vitamin C, betaine and methionine.

Acetylation Support

Acetylation depends on vitamin C, thiamine (B1) and pantothenic acid (B5).

Bile Synthesis Support

Bile is produced by the liver to break down fats in the intestine, act as a "detergent" and to carry toxins with it that are produced by the liver. Bile production and flow must be optimal for detoxification. Taurine, vitamin C, betaine (beet root), lecithin (phosphatidylcholine), methionine, inositol and l-carnitine have been shown to support bile production and flow.

I use many different detoxification programs depending on each individual case. Detoxification can be a vital part of optimizing thyroid function due to the multiple thyroid disruptors in our environment. Be sure to be adequately evaluated by a qualified functional medicine practitioner before beginning a detoxification program. A properly performed detoxification program should not result in sickness or severe symptoms.

CHAPTER FIVE
The Thyroid-Adrenal-Pancreas Axis

In addition to gastrointestinal and blood sugar disorders, adrenal gland dysfunction is the most commonly seen imbalance in today's society. Adrenal gland imbalances are also one of the major factors that cause thyroid hormone imbalance. Stress from work, relationships, electronics, poor diet choices such as consumption of refined carbohydrates and trans fats, infections, and environmental toxins all contribute to adrenal disorders.

The Adrenal Glands
The adrenal glands are about the size of a walnut and lie on top of the kidneys. The outer adrenal cortex comprises eighty percent of the gland and produces many hormones including cortisol and DHEA from cholesterol. Ninety percent of the cholesterol in the body is made by the liver and only ten percent comes from the diet. Cholesterol converts into the hormone pregnenolone in

the adrenal cortex which then converts to cortisol, the stress hormone, or DHEA, the sex hormone source, immune enhancer and anabolic. Cortisol is our "fight or flight" stress hormone. Cortisol slows down digestion, suppresses immune function and raises blood sugar as a survival mechanism when we are under stress. The problem arises when this becomes chronic and over time, elevated cortisol will tear down your body. Cortisol is secreted on a circadian rhythm with highest production in the morning that slowly tapers off as the day progresses. Sleep is when our bodies repair and rejuvenate but high cortisol during sleep will prevent this from happening.

Hormones Secreted by the Adrenal Glands

DHEA

DHEA (dehydroepiandrosterone) is a precursor to estrogens, progesterone and testosterone. DHEA is extremely important for immune system function and anabolic (building up) processes in the body. DHEA levels begin to decline after age thirty-five but cortisol can remain elevated during continuing periods of stress. Low DHEA levels are also found in diseases such as multiple sclerosis, cancer, fibromyalgia, lupus, rheumatoid arthritis, Crohn's, ulcerative colitis and of course, thyroid disorders.

Healthy adrenal glands are required for the conversion of inactive T4 into active T3.

When the adrenals have reached a state of fatigue, they are no longer producing sufficient cortisol or DHEA. This leaves individuals more susceptible to chronic diseases from an inability to compensate for the stresses they encounter on a daily basis. It is very important to treat the adrenal glands before commencing treatment of the thyroid. Increasing thyroid hormone production while the adrenals are in fatigue can overwhelm the adrenals and lead to further exhaustion. I have found that once the adrenal glands are healthy and the other related system/factors associated with thyroid imbalance are optimized, there is no need to treat the thyroid directly.

The inner medulla produces adrenalin and noradrenalin also known as norepinephrine and epinephrine. The cortex is under the control of hormones produced in the brain and the medulla is under the control of the nervous system.

Healthy adrenal glands are vital for women who are peri- and post-menopausal. The adrenal glands are responsible for producing the majority of sex hormones in a menopausal woman once the ovaries stop functioning. If the adrenal glands are fatigued and not ready for menopause, there will be an exaggeration of menopausal symptoms such as hot flashes, weight gain, sleep problems, bone loss, mood swings, depression, anxiety, loss of sex drive and vaginal dryness. Healthy adrenals ensure an easy transition into menopause and beyond. A vast majority of the women I see in practice approach menopause with adrenal fatigue leading to severe menopausal symptoms and hormone dysfunction.

Aldosterone

Aldosterone is produced by the cortex and causes sodium absorption and potassium excretion. Low salt diets and high water intake put a major stress on the adrenal glands to retain as much salt as possible as the blood becomes more diluted from the extra water intake. One of the easiest ways to maintain healthy adrenals is to consume a half- teaspoon of unrefined celtic sea salt every morning with a few glasses of water. It's important to consume half of your bodyweight in ounces of water every day but it must be balanced with salt to remove stress from the adrenal glands.

Cortisol

Cortisol is also produced by the cortex which increases blood sugar when it is low or if the body is under stress. Cortisol will cause glucose production in the liver or it will strip muscle tissue of protein to make glucose. Excess cortisol over long periods of time can increase the risk of diabetes due to prolonged blood sugar elevations.

Adrenaline

Adrenaline produced by the adrenal medulla will also raise blood sugar if there is stress on the body. Adrenaline will also increase fat circulation so that it can be burned as energy. This is not a good scenario for someone who is sitting at a desk and under major stress. Large amounts of fat and sugar floating in the bloodstream should be utilized to run from a saber-toothed tiger which is our built-in survival mechanism. If there is no activity, the excess sugar will be converted into fat and stored mainly around the mid-section, hips and thighs.

The adrenal cortex communicates with the pituitary gland and hypothalamus in the brain. The hypothalamus reads the amount of circulating hormones and tells the pituitary to make hormones that directly tell the cortex to make hormones. This is called the HPA axis or hypothalamic-pituitary-adrenal axis.

All hormones are secreted on a circadian rhythm over a 24-hour period. Cortisol is especially representative of this rhythm as cortisol production is the highest in the early morning and then slowly tapers off as the day progresses. Cortisol levels are lowest at night so that the body can repair itself to the best of its ability. You lose two-thirds of your stored sugar while sleeping and cortisol production ensures balanced blood sugar during the night. If the adrenals are fatigued, you may have trouble staying asleep as the body will make adrenaline to raise blood sugar due to inadequate cortisol production which is enough to wake you up. If your adrenals are in overdrive with too much cortisol production, then you probably have trouble falling asleep. If you are a slow starter in the morning, your adrenals are probably fatigued and can't make adequate cortisol to raise blood sugar and get you going in the morning.

The adrenals will go through phases of adaptation to stress beginning with elevated cortisol due to the initial stress. In the second stage, the adrenals will begin to use sex hormone precursors to make cortisol and DHEA will drop. The final stage is adrenal exhaustion/fatigue when the adrenals can no longer produce cortisol and DHEA. If you have adrenal gland dysfunction you may have the following symptoms:

Can't fall asleep
Can't stay asleep
Fatigue
Salt or sugar cravings
Allergies
Slow to start in the morning
Headaches
Weakened immune system
Ulcers
Need to eat to relieve fatigue
Irritable before meals
Shaky or lightheaded if meals are missed
Blurred vision
Crave caffeine or cigarettes
Feeling full or bloated
Dizziness
Asthma

Varicose veins
Hemorrhoids

Remember that the hormone aldosterone made in the adrenal cortex regulates blood volume through sodium retention and potassium excretion. If you have the following symptoms you have low aldosterone levels indicating adrenal gland dysfunction:

Craving salt
Fluid retention in the arms and legs
Pupils do not stay constricted when exposed to light
Rough or sandpaper tongue
Excessive urination – up to 15-20 times/day
Excessive sweating even without activity

Your natural physician will order a salivary hormone profile to measure cortisol production at four different times throughout the day. This allows your physician to observe adrenal gland dysfunction during all parts of the day and will dictate the type of treatment you will receive. Symptoms cannot adequately diagnose if the adrenals are in fatigue or if they are hyperfunctioning. This is why testing is so vital to properly assess adrenal gland function. In addition, it gives a baseline to compare to follow-up testing so treatment can be adjusted accordingly.

Blood sugar is intricately related to adrenal gland function and vice versa. Chronically elevated cortisol levels from adrenal stress will cause insulin receptor insensitivity. This basically means that when insulin binds to cell receptors to allow glucose (blood sugar) entry into the cell, the receptors may not respond which leaves sugar floating in the blood stream. Remember that excess sugar will be converted into fat and stored mainly around the abdomen, hips and thighs. This also puts extra stress on the pancreas to make more insulin to deal with the excess blood sugar which increases the risk of diabetes. As discussed earlier, cortisol is very important for blood sugar stability.

Hypoglycemia is a condition in which there is inadequate cortisol to raise blood sugar into the normal range. We usually see adrenal fatigue and hypoglycemia together. Hypoglycemics develop symptoms of low blood sugar and need to eat something to normalize blood sugar levels. They may feel shaky, irritable, light-headed, fatigued or may crave sugar because their adrenal glands cannot raise blood sugar into the normal range. Once hypoglycemics rejuvenate their adrenal glands, the symptoms will subside. It's important for hypoglycemics to eat frequently throughout the day and not skip meals. Each meal should be a combination of protein, carbohydrates and fats as a low-carb meal or too many carbs will further throw off blood sugar levels.

You may ask which comes first – adrenal dysfunction or blood sugar dysfunction? It doesn't matter because when one starts to become imbalanced so goes the other. This is also important to understand in treatment because both aspects should be addressed at the same time for optimal results.

So how does all this relate to optimal thyroid function? In the chapter on thyroid hormone physiology, we discussed the enzyme that converts inactive T4 (thyroxine) into active T3 (triiodothyronine). Remember that 93 percent of the hormone produced by the thyroid is inactive T4 until it is activated mainly in the liver by an enzyme. Cortisol directly inhibits this enzyme (5'-deiodinase) which converts inactive T4 into active T3. This in part can lead to low T3 levels. In addition, elevated cortisol will cause thyroid hormone receptor insensitivity meaning that even if T3 levels are adequate, they may not be able to bind normally to receptor sites. Cortisol will also increase the production of reverse T3 which is inactive. Cortisol can also lower the levels of protein that binds to thyroid hormone so it can circulate in a stable structure. Iodine, as you know from a previous chapter, is extremely vital to thyroid health but high levels of cortisol will increase the excretion of iodide from the kidney. And finally, elevated cortisol will inhibit TSH (thyroid-stimulating hormone) production by disrupting hypothalamic-pituitary feedback leading to suboptimal TSH production in the range of 1.0-1.5. Has your physician adequately assessed your adrenals before treatment? It is very irresponsible for any physician to treat thyroid hormone dysfunction without thoroughly assessing adrenal gland physiology and of course, blood sugar.

Regarding cortisol's effect on thyroid hormones, Werner and Ingbar's The Thyroid: A Fundamental and Clinical Text, (8th edition), states: "Serum TSH, TBG (thyroid-binding protein), T4 and T3 concentrations are slightly decreased, albeit usually within the respective ranges of normal; serum free T4 values are normal."[11]

As discussed in our chapter on the liver, impaired detoxification can lead to abnormal thyroid function. Again, the adrenals come into play because elevated cortisol inhibits proper liver detoxification. It is sometimes necessary to support liver detoxification pathways while treating the adrenal glands and thyroid to optimize results and metabolize toxins, excess hormones and thyroid-disrupting chemicals. Signs of impaired liver detoxification include nausea, constipation, bloating, lack of response to treatment, acne, acne during menstrual cycle, medication sensitivity, and pale skin upon pressure.

I dedicated an entire chapter to the Gut-Thyroid connection. There is also a powerful Adrenal-Gut connection as well. Elevated cortisol levels slowly eat away at the immune system that lines the gastrointestinal (GI) tract. Cortisol also increases inflammation in the GI tract and prevents the cells that line the GI tract from regenerating which increases the risk of ulcers. This leads to increased infections from parasites, yeast, mold, fungi, viruses, and bacteria which further stresses the adrenal glands creating a vicious cycle. Leaky gut is another consequence of chronically elevated cortisol levels which is a condition in which gaps open in the intestinal barrier allowing undigested proteins and toxins to enter the bloodstream uninhibited. This puts a major stress on the body's immune system and can lead to immune dysfunction, adrenal stress, chronic fatigue and thyroid hormone imbalance.

Adrenals that are functioning at a low level tend to exhibit various symptoms and patterns. Adrenal-fatigued people usually have to run on caffeine and sugar throughout the day to keep going. They are dragging out of bed and say, "I need my coffee before I can do anything." This is a sad state because it indicates an extremely unhealthy individual who requires a legal drug just to function. These individuals crave sweets and crash many times throughout the day, especially in the afternoon, and need a "pick me up" such as another cup of coffee or something sweet. This further drives blood sugar and hormone imbalances leading to weight gain, insomnia, fatigue and an underactive thyroid gland. In addition, these people can usually fall asleep without problems but will wake up during the night. This happens because there is inadequate cortisol production to stabilize blood sugar so the adrenals release adrenaline instead which raises blood sugar but is also too stimulatory resulting in waking up and insomnia.

People with adrenal hyperfunctioning usually cannot fall asleep because there is too much cortisol production which has an excitatory effect on the nervous system. There are many possible causes of elevated cortisol that lead to too much cortisol production and eventually adrenal fatigue. The following cause adrenal stress:

Anemia – *red blood cells cannot deliver oxygen to body tissues*

Blood sugar imbalances
Low cholesterol – *statin medications such as Lipitor, Crestor, Zocor, etc.*
Infections
Gums
Urinary tract
Gastrointestinal
Mold, yeast or fungus
Lyme Disease/Tick-Borne Infections
Chronic virus
Dehydration – especially in athletes or those who fly frequently (it is *important to drink half of bodyweight in ounces of water every day*)
Poor dietary habits *(skipping meals, high intake of simple carbohydrates, etc.)*
Eating foods you are sensitive/allergic to
Leaky gut
Liver detoxification issues
Essential fatty acid deficiencies
Not enough sleep
Overexercise
Emotional stressors *(usually severe)*
Heavy metals
Autoimmune adrenals
Chronic use of SSRIs *(selective serotonin reuptake inhibitors, Prozac, etc.)*
Chronic pain
Environmental toxin exposures – *damages mitochondria*
Surgical menopause
Chronic tissue injury or inflammation *(autoimmune condition)*

It takes a great deal of time and effort to do the proper detective work to find out why someone is ill. The supplements covered at the end of this chapter are meant to complement diet and lifestyle changes. In order for a treatment plan to be successful, it is very important that the following guidelines are adhered to without deviation.

Adrenal stimulants will disrupt your treatment plan and consist of the following:

> **Inadequate sleep**
> **Eating sugar/simple carbohydrates**
> **Caffeine and decaffeinated beverages**
> **Nicotine**
> **Alcohol**
> **Food allergies**
> **Trans fats** (*hydrogenated or partially-hydrogenated oils*)
> **Artificial sweeteners**
> **Excess exercise**

As long as blood sugar levels are out of balance, it will be extremely difficult to restore proper adrenal function. Practice the following guidelines to ensure stable blood sugar levels:

> *Always eat breakfast that includes more protein than carbohydrates*
> *Eat every two to three hours*
> *Snack on protein and fat such as nuts, eggs and seeds*
> *Do not drink juice – this includes ALL juices which are nothing more than plant sugar*
> *Consume protein at every meal*

Blood sugar imbalances and a condition known as insulin

resistance are major factors in optimizing thyroid and adrenal health. Insulin resistance basically means that insulin receptors are no longer able to respond to insulin. Insulin binds to receptors and allows blood sugar to enter cells. With insulin resistance, insulin's effects are negated leaving excess blood sugar. The following symptoms can indicate insulin resistance:

Fatigue
Sugar cravings
Abdominal obesity
High blood pressure
Inability to lose weight
Always feeling hungry
Fatigue after meals
Aches and pains all over
High cholesterol, glucose, and triglycerides
Low HDL *("good" cholesterol)*

Remember that impaired liver detoxification can significantly affect optimal thyroid hormone function. Elevated insulin levels will reduce glutathione levels inhibiting the liver's ability to detoxify. This will affect the conversion of inactive T4 into active T3, increase thyroid-disrupting chemicals and may lead to excess estrogen levels which inhibit thyroid hormone function.

As discussed in the chapter on thyroid hormone basics, thyroid hormone's main function is to regulate metabolism through the burning of sugar, fat and protein. Insulin resistance prevents adequate sugar transport into the cell decreasing the available fuel for energy production. This puts an increased strain on the thyroid to make more hormone and can eventually lead to hypothyroidism.

We have already discussed the importance of adrenal gland

function and its relationship to optimal thyroid health. The following supplements will help to correct adrenal gland dysfunction. It's very important to have the adrenal hormones cortisol and DHEA tested to ensure precise treatment. Adaptogens are compounds that help to normalize the hypothalamic-pituitary-adrenal axis. They will help adrenals that are in a state of fatigue, high stress or a combination of both. The feedback loop of the HPA axis is key in balancing adrenal hormones, and adaptogens are vital in healing this process.

Supplements That Help Correct Adrenal Gland Dysfunction

Magnolia & Phellodendron
Magnolia is a tree native to the rain forests of China. Its bark has been used for a variety of medicinal purposes including the regulation of stress and anxiety. Phellodendron grows in northeastern China and Japan. Together, these extracts restore cortisol and DHEA production in the adrenal gland. They bind to stress hormone receptors promoting relaxation and feelings of well-being.

Perilla oil & MCTs
These essential oils have natural stress-reducing effects. Perilla oil is rich in omega-3 fatty acids which stimulate repair and are anti-inflammatory. MCTs reduce cell acids and help to produce energy in the cell's mitochondria. MCTs are easy to assimilate and metabolize which is extremely important for those with delicate stomachs and impaired absorption.

Ashwagandha
Ashwagandha is an adaptogen that is similar to panax ginseng. It has the ability to normalize adrenal stress syndromes. Stress responses can have many adverse affects on health and this herb will

reduce these effects.

Eleutherococcus

Eleutherococcus senticosus is an adaptogen that supports the HPA axis under times of stress as well as enhance athletic performance. Eleutherococcus will enhance physical work capacity as well as brain function when under stress.

Panax Ginseng

Panax ginseng is also known as Korean ginseng and is an adaptogen. Panax ginseng optimizes the functioning of the HPA axis. It has been shown to enhance physical performance, stamina and energy production. Panax ginseng will shift metabolism into a fat-burning state as opposed to a sugar-burning state due to an increase in oxygen availability for muscles.

Rhodiola

Rhodiola is popular in traditional Eastern European and Asian medical systems. Rhodiola is an adaptogen that has been shown to enhance immune function and brain function. It also has antidepressant properties, protects the heart and protects against cancer. Rhodiola will prevent adrenaline roller coasters due to high stress.

Holy Basil

Holy basil is an adaptogen that reduces cortisol production from stress, supports blood sugar, has antihistamine properties, optimizes the functioning of the HPA axis, improves the integrity of the gastrointestinal mucosal barrier, improves immune function, and enhances athletic performance.

Pantethine

Pantethine is required for adrenal hormone production. However, it will not over-stimulate cortisol production under times of stress but has the opposite effect.

Licorice (Glycyrrhiza Glabara)

Licorice contains compounds that increase the half-life of cortisol which removes stress on the adrenal glands to produce more cortisol. It also has been shown to boost the immune system, reduce inflammation and also reduce/minimize allergic responses. Licorice is antibacterial and antiviral. Due to estrogen's negative effect on thyroid function, licorice is of great benefit because it helps normalize estrogen metabolism.

PregnenolonePregnenolone is the "mother of all hormones" and is made from cholesterol in the adrenal gland. Pregnenolone converts into cortisol, DHEA, testosterone, estrogen and progesterone. Pregnenolone is a powerful antioxidant and has been shown to boost mood, improve memory and optimize brain function.

DHEA

DHEA is made by the adrenal glands and will convert into estrogen and testosterone. In men, it will mainly convert into estrogen and in women, DHEA will mainly convert into testosterone. DHEA has its own effects including resensitizing insulin receptors, boosting the immune system, preventing bone loss, enhancing memory and lowering cholesterol. When under stress, the body will make cortisol at the expense of DHEA.

Phosphatidylserine

Phosphatidylserine's greatest benefit is its ability to lower cortisol levels by optimizing the brain's relationship with the adrenal glands. After only ten days of high doses of PS, research has shown that excessive cortisol levels can be decreased in healthy men. PS has also been shown to enhance brain function and memory, decrease anxiety and depression, improve mood, and enhance metabolism. It is also an antioxidant. It is very difficult for the body to make PS as it requires many nutrients for production. Supplementation is vital for optimizing adrenal function so cortisol cannot have its negative effects on the body and the thyroid.

Supplements that Balance Blood Sugar

Blood sugar imbalances will greatly influence the ability of your thyroid to function optimally. The following supplements are vital in balancing blood sugar.

Huckleberry/Bilberry (Vaccinium myrtillus)

The extract from the leaves of this plant has been shown to lower blood sugar levels and has been used traditionally to treat diabetes.

Galega Officinalis (French lilac)

This plant has been utilized since the Middle Ages in the treatment of diabetes. French lilac lowers blood sugar by decreasing insulin resistance. Prescription medications for blood sugar control such as Metformin are derived from the active ingredients in French lilac.

Gymnema Sylvestre

Gymnema sylvestre has been shown to regenerate the beta cells in the pancreas that produce insulin. This herb will enhance the effects of insulin, reduce fasting blood sugar, decrease the need for insulin and help with insulin resistance. It will not cause a state of hypoglycemia, however.

Chromium

Chromium stabilizes blood sugar and insulin levels after meals.

It will also ensure optimal delivery of blood sugar into your cells. Deficiencies in this nutrient can lead to insulin resistance, high cholesterol and abnormalities in sugar's ability to bind to red blood cells.

Zinc

Zinc's role in blood sugar management includes optimizing insulin metabolism, protecting insulin-producing beta cells of the pancreas and improving insulin sensitivity which ensures optimal uptake of sugar into your cells.

Vanadium

Vanadium is very important for insulin resistance by improving transport of sugar into your cells due to its insulin-like effects on cell receptors.

Alpha lipoic acid (ALA)

ALA is another important nutrient for insulin resistance and is also a strong antioxidant. ALA increases energy production by your cells, optimizes sugar metabolism and lowers lactic acid levels.

Vitamin E

Vitamin E should not be taken in its alpha tocopherol form. Mixed tocopherols including gamma and delta tocopherol are the preferred form of delivery. Vitamin E improves insulin sensitivity, lowers blood fats, is a powerful antioxidant and lowers the so-called "bad" LDL cholesterol.

Biotin

Biotin is important in supporting the liver's utilization of sugar. This nutrient will enhance insulin's effects as well as lower blood sugar levels after meals.

Magnesium

Entire books have been written on the king of minerals. Magnesium is involved in approximately 350 reactions in the body and deficiencies in our society are rampant. Magnesium deficiency will lead to insulin resistance and abnormal sugar metabolism. Magnesium appears to enhance insulin secretion by the pancreas.

L-carnitine

L-carnitine is a di-peptide compound that shuttles fatty acids in the cell to be burned as energy. Carnitine has similar effects on blood sugar by supporting sugar transport into cells.

CHAPTER SIX
Hormone-Thyroid Connection

Testosterone

Testosterone is made in the testes and adrenal glands in a male, and in a woman, the ovaries and adrenal glands. Testosterone is very important for metabolism. It has been shown that low thyroid states result in low testosterone levels. When the thyroid gland returns to optimal function in individuals with challenged thyroids, their testosterone levels also return to normal. Testosterone replacement can help many conditions including thyroid and autoimmune diseases but simply giving these patients testosterone without correcting the reason why their testosterone is low in the first place does a great disservice to these patients in the long run. Testosterone replacement suppresses the pituitary hormone that signals the testes to make testosterone. Once the patient comes off of the testosterone, one's natural production may be suppressed resulting in dependence on the prescribing physician for continued hormone replacement. There are a variety of factors that must be addressed before prescribing testosterone which should be done as a last resort. It is very "sexy" in this day and age to get bioidentical hormones which are of course superior to synthetic hormones but still do not address underlying imbalances. The following must be addressed before commencing testosterone replacement:

> **Liver detoxification**
> **Estrogen metabolism**
> **GI microflora activity**
> **Insulin sensitivity**
> **Adrenal function**
> **Testosterone synthesis**
> **5-alpha reductase activity** *(converts testosterone into di-hydrotestosterone)*
> **Beta-glucuronidase activity**
> **17,20 lyase activity**–*progesterone to androstenedione*
> **Aromatase activity**
> **Hypothalamic-Pituitary feedback loops**

Progesterone

Progesterone is mainly produced during the second half of a woman's menstrual cycle. It is manufactured mainly in the ovaries and some in the adrenal glands in women. In men, it is made in the adrenals and testes. Progesterone enhances thyroid hormone function but a low thyroid can result in inadequate progesterone production. Like all other hormones, progesterone should not be used for long periods of time and should be used in minimal doses. Progesterone creams bypass the intestinal tract and liver which is more desirable than pills or sublingual drops. Many women use progesterone cream based on symptoms which many times does more harm than good. You should always have your hormone levels tested first before using hormone replacment. Synthetic progesterone known as Provera, Depo-Provera, etc. has been shown to increase the risk of breast cancer by 800%. Synthetic progesterone is not actually the progesterone that your body makes but a chemically-modified form of progesterone.

Estrogen

Estrogen is made in the ovaries in cycling women but the majority of estrogen in a menopausal woman is made in the adrenal gland. There are three types of estrogen:

Estrone or E1–10%
Estradiol or E2–10%
Estriol or E3–80%

The percentages indicate the amount that is naturally produced in the body. Synthetic estrogens are given in very high doses of estrone or estradiol with little to no amount of estriol throwing off the natural balance of estrogen in a woman's body. This is one of the reasons why the Women's Health Initiative was stopped before its completion due to the many side effects.

Estrogen is important for healthy bones, brain function, sex drive and function and may have a protective effect from heart disease. As with any hormone, too much estrogen can have negative effects, especially an increased risk of breast cancer. We are living in an estrogen-dominant world due to the many chemicals that act like estrogen known as xenoestrogens.

Elevated estrogen can be due to stress, diet, exposure to xenoestrogens and impaired hormone detoxification systems. Stress will actually free inactive estrogen to active estrogen leading to side effects such as water retention, breast cysts, moodiness, and weight gain. Conventional meat from animals injected with estrogen can be a problem as well. The excess estrogen in the animals leads to weight gain from water retention increasing profits due to

more money per pound. Fiber, liver detoxification, stress reduction and the elimination of conventional dairy and meat in the diet
will lower excess estrogen.

We know that excess estrogen can lead to low thyroid function.
The mechanism behind this is simply an inhibition of the conversion of inactive T4 into active T3 as well as estrogen binding to the
proteins to which thyroid hormone would normally bind.

Women who are taking synthetic estrogens such as Premarin,
Prempro and the birth control pill will most likely have low thyroid function due to the excess estrogen. Many times, cleansing
the body of excess estrogen and ensuring proper estrogen metabolism in the liver can clear the symptoms of hypothyroidism.

It is a very rare case where we will use estrogen in our practice
due to the fact that correcting underlying physiology can normalize estrogen levels. This is also true for post-menopausal women
who usually have low estrogen due to concomitant adrenal fatigue. When the adrenal glands are healthy in a post-menopausal
woman, she will usually have adequate estrogen in her system.

Pregnenolone
Pregnenolone or "the mother of all hormones" is made from cholesterol mainly in the adrenal glands. As its name suggests, it is
the precursor to all of your sex hormones including testosterone,
estrogen, progesterone, DHEA and cortisol. Pregnenolone is
found in its highest concentration in the brain and is important for
memory and brain function. Research has shown that those with
low thyroid function also have low pregnenolone levels. We use
time-released pregnenolone in our patients with adrenal fatigue to
rebuild the adrenal glands when they are exhausted. Most of the
pregnenolone taken will convert into cortisol which is good if the
adrenal glands are exhausted and not producing enough cortisol.
Remember that too much cortisol inhibits thyroid function but on

the flip side you need some cortisol to convert inactive T4 into active T3. Patients tend to notice an instant increase in energy and memory and have an improved sense of well-being once they begin taking pregnenolone.

DHEA

DHEA is a steroid hormone produced in the adrenal gland. There is plenty of research showing that patients with low DHEA levels also have low thyroid function. Like pregnenolone, DHEA is given to our patients who have adrenal fatigue to rebuild the adrenals. DHEA is not taken for long periods of time, however, as it can cause hormonal imbalances if not taken correctly. DHEA has its own effects in the body including proper immune function, fat burning, muscle building, tissue repair, proper liver function and energy production. DHEA will also convert into other sex hormones such as estrogen and testosterone. When DHEA is given to a woman, it will most likely convert into testosterone but in a man it will most likely convert into estrogen. DHEA received a lot of press as an anti-aging hormone which led to abuse of its over-the-counter availability. DHEA should not be taken without proper testing first and it should be taken in the lowest dose possible.

Cortisol

Cortisol is made in the adrenal gland to raise blood sugar into the normal range but chronic elevations of cortisol can lead to blood sugar problems. Cortisol in high doses is a catabolic hormone meaning it breaks down the body's tissues. Cortisol also eats away at the area of the brain that is involved in memory known as the hippocampus. Cortisol is also required for an adequate immune response to infection so if you have trouble recovering from infections you may have inadequate adrenal gland function. Cortisol converts into cortisone which is your body's natural anti-inflammatory. Too much cortisol will suppress TSH (thyroid-stimulating hormone), inhibit the conversion of inactive T4 into active T3 and also directly block thyroid hormone receptors. Cortisol is required, however, to convert inactive T4 into active T3 making it very important for proper thyroid hormone function.

The adrenal glands should nearly always be treated before the thyroid is treated due to the fact that too much thyroid hormone can make already fatigued adrenals even worse. I have also found that once the adrenals are functioning optimally, many patients' thyroid symptoms resolve indicating it was not a thyroid problem in the first place.

CHAPTER SEVEN
Thyroid-Disrupting Chemicals

With approximately 100,000 chemicals in commercial use today and approximately 4,000-6,000 new chemicals produced each year, it is no wonder we are becoming so sick.12-13 Eighty percent of these chemicals have never been tested for human safety or their effects on the unborn.[14]

There are many chemicals known as thyroid-disrupting chemicals (TDCs) that can also be classified as endocrine-disrupting chemicals. These chemicals can affect normal production of thyroid hormone, its circulating levels in the blood and can harm hormone receptors preventing hormones from binding and doing their job. These chemicals have received more press as of late due to their effect on the developing brain leading to impaired cognitive function and behavioral problems. Thyroid hormone directly affects genetic expression requiring proper communication within each cell. It is thus hypothesized that TDCs can alter gene expression.

Polychlorinated biphenyls, polybrominated diphenyl ethers, polybrominated biphenyls, phthalates, bisphenol-A and halogens such as fluoride, bromide and iodide can bind to thyroid hormone receptors and exert negative effects. Thyroid hormone is extremely important for brain development. We are literally poisoning our children with chemicals that impair brain function.

It has been shown that chemical exposure can lead to low circulating levels of thyroid hormone as well as altered thyroid hormone metabolism. One possible scenario that can occur is normal thyroid hormone blood tests but symptoms of low thyroid function due to chemical binding to thyroid receptors altering their affinity for thyroid hormone. Your thyroid may be producing adequate amounts of thyroid hormone but with multiple poisoned receptors not responding to thyroid hormone, your doctor will tell you that you are fine when you really aren't.

One example is PCBs or polychlorinated biphenyls which are abundant in our environment even though they were banned in the 1970s. They are still found in high concentrations in human tissues and have a high affinity for the brain. Infants that are only six-weeks-old have been found to have elevated levels of PCBs. Most of this comes from breast milk as bottle-fed babies do not have levels as high as breastfed babies. But what do the bottle-fed babies have more of? This high exposure to the developing brain leaves many children extremely vulnerable to impaired brain development and impaired thyroid function.

Studies have shown that early exposure to PCBs results in neuropsychological deficits such as low IQ, attention deficit disorder, impaired coordination and reduced ability to remember what has been seen. These negative effects are due to PCBs binding to thyroid hormone receptors and altering their function. PCBs have also been shown to lower circulating levels of T4 (thyroxine) in rats.

Bisphenol-A (BPA) is produced at approximately 800 million

kg every year in the US mainly to be used in the manufacturing of plastics including resins that coat food cans, dental sealants and polycarbonate plastics.[15] Resin-lined food cans contribute a large source of human consumption of Bisphenol-A. BPA has been found in the blood of pregnant women, in the amniotic fluid, and in the umbilical cord after birth as well as the placenta. BPA can also be chemically altered to make flame retardants by adding bromine or chlorine which are known thyroid disrupters. The most common is tetrabromobisphenol-A or TBBPA which is a flame retardant produced at about 60,000 tons annually.[16] Its levels have increased in human blood since 1977.[17]

BPA has been specifically shown to bind to thyroid receptors and can be considered a weak estrogen. When BPA binds to a thyroid receptor, it directly inhibits binding of the active thyroid hormone T3. This could lead to another example of normal thyroid hormone levels but all the symptoms of hypothyroidism in a person. One study found that rats exposed to BPA developed attention-deficit hyperactivity disorder.[18]

Polybrominated diphenyl ether (PBDE) is an emerging chemical that is a flame retardant and is being found in greater concentrations in human tissues. Triclosan is a chemical with similar structure and has been shown to interfere with thyroid hormone receptors. Triclosan is used as an antibacterial agent in soaps and creams and has been found in human blood.

There are many more chemicals out there, but these are the most heavily researched regarding their effects on thyroid hormone and thyroid receptors. We are all exposed to these chemicals on a daily basis but we can limit the exposure and follow specific detoxification programs to rid them from our body's tissues. Eliminate use of plastics as much as possible and use glass or stainless steel bottles to carry your water. Do not use products that have flame retardants and don't buy carpeting that is treated with such chemicals. Do not use antibacterial products which shouldn't be used for other reasons such as their ability to kill beneficial bacteria on the skin. Periodically cleanse your body following a physician-supervised program to ensure optimal detoxification and to prevent reabsorption of toxins.

Over the past decade, there has been increasing evidence that toxic chemicals can disrupt hormone synthesis including sex hormones such as testosterone and estrogen. We now know that these chemicals can significantly affect thyroid function as well as thyroid hormone once it is produced. These chemicals can affect thyroid hormone production, hormone receptors, cellular uptake mechanisms, thyroid hormone metabolism and transport proteins that bind to thyroid hormone. Some chemicals even have structural resemblance to thyroid hormone T4 and T3 thus having the effect of binding to receptor sites and inducing hypothyroid symptoms even when blood testing reveals normal levels.

Polychlorinated biphenyls (PCBs)

There are approximately 209 PCBs which accumulate in fatty tissue and have structural resemblance to T4 (thyroxine) which is the main hormone produced by the thyroid gland.[19] PCBs have been shown to reduce circulating levels of thyroid hormones including T4, free T4, and total T3, and increase TSH. Mothers who are exposed to PCBs will transfer these chemicals to the fetus; this chemical has actually been found in fetal brain, liver and plasma. Total T4 and free T4 levels were found to be decreased and TSH increased in fetal blood samples. PCB77 specifically reduced thyroid hormone levels in the fetus. One study found that adults, adolescents and children from areas of high PCB exposure also had decreased levels of circulating thyroid hormones. Another study was done to assess thyroid volume of those living in areas of high PCB exposure. Thyroid ultrasounds of the subjects revealed significantly larger thyroids than in non-exposed individuals.

Unfortunately, these chemicals not only affect humans but have also been shown to significantly reduce T3 and T4 levels in sea lions, polar bears and seals.

Dioxins

Dioxins aka polychlorinated dibenzo-p-dioxin (PCDDs), TCDD (most toxic) and furans (PCDFs) are highly toxic chemicals from the production of herbicides and industrial burning processes. TCDDs were given to pregnant rats and were found in their offspring by route of not only transplacental delivery but also through breastfeeding. A single dose of TCDDs resulted in decreased T4, free T4, and increased TSH as well as increased size of the thyroid glands. In humans, TCDDs resulted in increased levels of TSH.

Flame Retardants

TBBPAs, PBDEs, PCBs and BPAs are extensively used flame retardants in plastics, paints, synthetic textiles, televisions, computers, copying machines, video displays and laser printers. PBDEs have been shown to reduce circulating thyroid hormone levels in rodents. In addition, they upregulated important liver detoxification enzymes and caused tissue changes in the thyroid gland indicating hypothyroidism.

Bromkal is a popular commercial mixture shown to reduce total and free T4 levels. Total T4 levels decrease in fish after exposure to PBDE. When pregnant rats were exposed to PBDE, their offspring had reduced levels of circulating thyroid hormones.

Phenols

Phenols include nonylphenol (NP), pentachlorophenol (PCP) and BPA. Phenols are industrial additives used in many detergents, pesticides and plastics. Phenols have also been used as antifungals, wood preservatives, biocides. BPA is used to manufacture plastic products such as polycarbonate water bottles, food can linings, compact discs, powder paints, adhesives and dental sealants. When rats are exposed to phenols, their TSH levels increase and T4 and T3 levels also actually increase indicating impaired thyroid hormone metabolism. In ewes, phenols decreased levels of circulating T4. Exposure to BPA in voles resulted in upregulation of liver detoxification enzymes indicating liver stress. In human newborns, PCP was found in spinal cord plasma with decreased levels of T3, free T4 and thyroid-binding globulin (a protein that transports T4).

Phthalates

Phthalates are chemicals found in plastics such as bottled water, food storage containers, and plastic food wraps (Saran wrap). They are also found in cosmetics and personal products including nail polish remover, hair spray, perfume and eye shadow. Even the popular glow sticks that children use are loaded with phthalates. Rodent studies have shown that exposure to phthalates resulted in tissue changes in the thyroid gland with resultant hyperactivity. Phthalates have varying effects on circulating thyroid hormones as some studies show they increase hormone levels and some show they decrease them.

Parabens

Parabens are widely used as a preservative in cosmetics, foods, and prescription drugs. Studies show that parabens have estrogen-like effects that can inhibit thyroid function as well as cause symptoms of excess estrogen. Methylparaben has been shown to have antithyroid activity by inhibiting iodine.

Pesticides

DDT and HCB are the most extensively studied of pesticides that affect the thyroid. DDT exposure has been shown to decrease T4 and increase the weight of the thyroid in birds. The more DDT that was found in the blubber of seals resulted in lower total T3 and free T3 levels. HCB has many studies showing that exposure decreases T4 and T3 levels. Even prenatal exposure reduced T4 and free T4 levels and upregulated enzymes that metabolize thyroid hormone in the fetal brain. Thyroid glands in humans enlarge when they are exposed to HCB which then causes a reduction of T4.

How Do Chemicals Inhibit Thyroid Function?

Each chemical affects thyroid function in its own unique way. Perchlorates work by inhibiting the uptake of iodine into the thyroid cells. Phthalates actually increase the uptake of iodine into the thyroid resulting in too much hormone production. Phenols inhibit the enzyme in the thyroid that is required to make thyroid hormone. DDT and PCB inhibit the function of TSH receptors. PCBs, phthalates, phenols, flame retardants and HCB have all been shown to bind to proteins that transport thyroid hormone which disrupts hormone binding and metabolism. Phthalates and chlordanes inhibit cellular uptake of thyroid hormones. PCBs, phenols, flame retardants, BPA and HCB all inhibit thyroid hormone receptors and inhibit gene expression in the cell. PCBs, dioxins, phenols, flame retardants, HCB and BPA all affect the metabolism/rate of excretion of thyroid hormones.

Humans are exposed to an increasing number of environmental chemicals on a daily basis. The research is clear that these can significantly disrupt thyroid function in many ways. There is a delicate balance between TSH and T4 physiology in the body and even a minute change in this balance can cause symptoms and even inhibit proper brain and nervous system development in children. This creates a serious issue for reasons that are too obvious to explore any further.

The Environmental Working Group at www.ewg.org has an excellent cosmetic database that provides information on many cosmetic products and the harmful chemicals that they contain. A search can be done on the website and each product is rated on a safety scale including detailed information on the negative effects of each chemical in the body.

CHAPTER EIGHT
Toxic Metals

Toxic metals can significantly inhibit thyroid gland and thyroid hormone function. Toxic metals inhibit thyroid hormone function by poisoning the enzyme that converts T4 into the more active T3. Toxic metals can also affect thyroid hormone receptors having a negative effect on even normal levels of thyroid hormone. They can be somewhat similar in effect to thyroid-disrupting chemicals as discussed in chapter seven. Toxic metals can also enter the energy-producing parts of your cells known as mitochondria and break down their ability to produce energy from fat and sugar-burning. Toxic metals accumulate in body tissues such as the thyroid, brain, heart, liver, pancreas, bone, etc. Some metals have a higher affinity for specific tissues. Mercury has the highest affinity for the thyroid. Listed below are the most significant toxic metals, where you can be exposed by them and the symptoms they cause.

Aluminum

Aluminum is found in beverage cans, pots and pans, foil, metal alloys, water treatment parts, furnace linings, antacids, antiperspirants, astringents, aspirin, food additives, dialysis, cosmetics and colloidal mineral products.

Symptoms of aluminum toxicity include: lung disease, bone softening, neurotoxicity, and possible Alzheimer's disease.

Arsenic

Arsenic is found in automobile batteries, asphalt, smelters, wood preservative, pesticides, insecticides, herbicides, glass, electronics, semiconductors, pigments, well water, seafood and shellfish, smog, rodent poisons and fungicides.

Symptoms of arsenic toxicity include: lung disease, decreased white blood cell production, anemia, birth defects, anxiety, cancer, heart arrhythmias, neurotoxicity, depression, garlic breath, headaches, hyperpigmentation of skin, keratosis, nerve pain/radiating pain, spontaneous abortion and kidney inflammation.

Cadmium

Cadmium is found in asphalt, batteries, metal plating, pigments, plastics, paints, metal soldering and welding, semiconductors, photography, printing, textiles, shellfish, liver and kidney meat, cigarette smoke, fertilizer, drinking water, fungicides, rubber and photoconductors.

Symptoms of cadmium toxicity include: lung disease, kidney toxicity, anemia, behavioral disorders, cancer, emphysema, headaches, high blood pressure, bone softening, autoimmune disease, depressed immune function, neurotoxicity, birth defects and infertility.

Lead

Lead is found in crystal, pesticides, batteries, solder, pipes, roofing materials, caulking, buckles, petroleum, radiation protection, pigments, paints, plastics, ceramics, electrical devices, tv glass, brass, bronze, gasoline, ammunition, electrical wire insulation, drinking water, fertilizer and candle wicks.

Symptoms of lead toxicity include: gastrointestinal problems, colic, anemia, neurotoxicity, nerve pain, liver toxicity, impaired liver detoxification, EKG abnormalities, infertility, inner ear toxicity, growth retardation, delayed development, impaired coordination, fatigue, anxiety, headaches, immune system toxicity and cancer.

Mercury

Mercury tends to be the most problematic toxic metal for the thyroid gland. An excellent paper was published in 2009 in Critical Reviews in Toxicology entitled, "The Endocrine Effects of Mercury in Humans and Wildlife." The authors state:

> *We concluded that there are five main mechanisms by which mercury influences the thyroid-adrenal and reproductive endocrine systems: (a) accumulation in the endocrine system; (b) specific cytotoxicity in endocrine tissues; (c) changes in hormonal concentrations; (d) interactions with sex hormones; and (e) up-regulation or down-regulation of enzymes within the steroidogenesis pathway.*

There are three main types of mercury that have been determined to have negative effects on humans and animals. They include methylmercury (MeHg), HgCl2 and elemental mercury (Hg2+). Methyl mercury is the type of mercury to which humans are mainly exposed.

The majority of mercury exposure comes from the burning of fossil fuels (coal) for power and the by-products of heating and waste incineration. Dental amalgams account for the largest percentage of non-occupational mercury exposure. Tuna, marlin and swordfish contain the highest levels of mercury (methylmercury) among fish. The smaller and younger the fish, the less mercury it will contain. Although mercury tends to accumulate mainly in the liver and kidneys, it also has a high affinity for the endocrine system including the thyroid gland. One study looked at mercury accumulation in mercury mine workers and found that mercury levels in the thyroid were three to four times higher than in the kidneys.[21]

Mercury has been shown to disrupt the Hypothalamic-Pituitary-Thyroid axis due to accumulation in all three glands. It has been shown that mercury exposure can either increase or decrease TSH levels. This is also true for T4, T3 and reverse T3. Mercury exposure also affects the gland itself causing an increase in size as well as increased rates thyroid cancer.

There are different ways in which mercury can affect thyroid function. Mercury can inhibit the thyroid peroxidase enzyme (TPO) which is required for thyroid hormone production. Iodine is required for the production of thyroid hormone as discussed in the iodine chapter. Mercury inhibits the uptake of iodine into the thyroid gland and also increases the rate that iodine is excreted from the body through the kidneys. Mercury binds to the main enzyme (5'-deiodinase) involved in the conversion of T4 to T3, altering its function. Selenium has a high affinity for mercury and will bind to it for removal from the body. Selenium has been shown to decrease the toxic effects of mercury but mercury exposure will rapidly deplete body stores of selenium. It is very important for those with mercury exposure to supplement with extra selenium to protect not only the thyroid but the rest of the body as well.

Mercury has also been shown to disrupt the Hypothalamic-Pituitary-Adrenal axis which is covered in detail in the adrenal and blood sugar chapter. Remember that healthy adrenals are critical for optimizing thyroid function. Mercury directly affects the hypothalamus and pituitary gland which are the masters of adrenal hormone production. Mercury also can disrupt that actual production of adrenal hormones as well as the pathways where hormones are formed. Like the thyroid, the adrenal glands also grow in size when exposed to mercury.

In addition to thyroid and adrenal hormones, mercury inhibits the conversion of cholesterol into pregnenolone (the mother of all hormones) and also disrupts steroid hormone production in the body. Most of the studies on mercury's effects on adrenal hormone production show that it decreases production of cortisol and aldosterone while spiking DHEA. Initially, mercury exposure can increase adrenaline and cortisol production due to the stress response from toxin exposure but over time, cortisol levels will drop.

Mercury is found in thermometers, batteries, fish, pigments, antibacterial products, antiseptic creams, skin lightening creams, fireworks, dental amalgams, pesticides, asphalt, agricultural chemicals, photography, taxidermy, electrical equipment, electroplating, felt, textiles, interior paint, hemorrhoidal preparations, hospital wastes, waste incineration, paper industry, explosives and fungicides.

Symptoms of mercury toxicity include: fatigue, neurotoxicity, emotional disturbances, nerve pain, altered sex drive, birth defects, spontaneous abortion, excessive salivation, tremors, irritability, menstrual disorders, autoimmune disease and kidney inflammation.

Nickel

Nickel is found in jewelry, coins, stainless steel, ceramics, pigments, cast iron, batteries, electroplating, metal alloys, electrical circuits, dyes, pesticides, asphalt, tobacco smoke, volcanoes, power plants, waste incinerators, diesel exhaust, cocoa and hydrogenated oils.

Symptoms of nickel toxicity include: dermatitis, respiratory irritation, cancer, emphysema, colic, excessive salivation, fatigue, headaches, muscle pain, vertigo, liver and kidney toxicity, and male infertility.

How do you get rid of toxic metals? There are many ways to do this and every doctor has his own way of doing it. Toxic metal elimination is an art and has no gold standard at this point. There are two basic theories on how to approach ridding them from the body. The first method is to simply support all of the detoxification systems of the body through diet, supplementation, and adjunctive modalities such as infrared saunas, colonics and salt and soda baths. The second method is to use chemical-based metal chelators such as DMSA, DMPS, d-penicillamine, and EDTA. A chelator is a substance that has a high affinity for metals and will bind to them to be excreted from the body. Both methods work wonders for patients but one method may work better than another for certain individuals. Some doctors who use metal chelators do not prepare the patient adequately for an intense heavy metal detox and the patient ends up becoming ill or has many side effects. The doctor then tells the patient that this is just a "detox reaction" to the treatment. It is very important to understand that any detoxification program should not make someone ill or have many side effects. If this happens, then the patient was not adequately prepared for the detox or there was not enough supportive nutrition as part of the program.

One example is detoxifying someone before her intestines are functioning optimally. If you have leaky gut syndrome then many of the toxins that are being dumped into the intestine from the liver/ gallbladder complex may reabsorb into the bloodstream and cause ill health and side effects. In addition, healthy bacterial colonies are required for the proper elimination of toxins through the intestinal tract. Certain minerals such as selenium are important because they bind to metals such as mercury making them inert so that they can be safely excreted in the feces.

Another important factor in preparation for detoxification and during the detox process is a sufficient amount of antioxidants. Detoxification can yield excessive free radical production increasing the need for antioxidants to neutralize the free radicals. Prior to detoxing and during detox, everyone should be sure their body is saturated with antioxidants.

As discussed in the liver and detoxification chapter, it is very important that both phases of liver detoxification are functioning optimally. This especially goes for phase 2 which can be very "delicate" in some individuals. Your genetics, nutritional status and environmental exposure determine how well these detox pathways are functioning. Some individuals require extra amino acids for phase 2 detoxification before beginning a detox program. I recommend the following for detox preparation:

Optimally functioning GI tract
Sufficient antioxidant saturation
Liver detoxification support
Alkaline Way diet *(ensure pH is alkaline before commencing program)*
Healthy immune system
Optimal amino acid reserves
No signs of inflammation

If these 7 are in place before beginning, you should not become sick or have many noticeable side effects from your program.

Testing for Metals

There are many different ways to test for toxic metals and some
are accurate and some are not. Hair analysis is not an accurate way
to test for toxic metal body burden. Hair analysis only shows you
what is being excreted in the hair. The problem with this method
is that some people do not excrete metals well through the hair and
some excrete metals very well through hair. If a test result shows
low metal excretion in hair, this means absolutely nothing as far
as how much metal is in the body. Also, a hair test that shows high
levels of metals can mean three things:

1. The patient has had recent high exposure to the
metal.
2. Genetically, the patient rapidly excretes metals
through the hair but may have low body burden.
3. The patient is currently going through a heavy
metal detox program.

So as you can see, the results from hair can be quite ambigu-
ous. The second way to test for metals is through blood testing.
The problem with blood is that once you are exposed to a toxic
metal, it is cleared from the blood within 72 hours and is excreted
or deposited in your tissues. If blood levels are high, then you can
assume that there was recent exposure to the metal. The third way
to test is in stool. This is a decent way to measure what is being
excreted through the liver/gallbladder complex but does not reflect
body burden. This is sometimes recommended for the very young
as it is easy to collect. The fourth and best way to test for metals
is a urine challenge test. This method is currently the most widely
used and accepted test for toxic metals. This is done by ingesting
or injecting a chelator such as DMSA, DMPS, d-penicillamine or
EDTA and then collecting the urine for two or six hours. This is

an excellent test because the chelators pull metals out of the body tissues which are then excreted in the urine. This gives us the best measure of toxic metal burden because it is a reflection of what is in the tissues. No test is totally accurate but the urine challenge test is the best we have right now.

Once it is known what metals are elevated through urine challenge testing, then a detox program can be tailor-made based on what metals are the most elevated. Repeat testing every two to three months is recommended to monitor progress.

The interesting thing about retesting metals is that sometimes a specific metal that was not elevated in the first test becomes elevated in the second or third test. You will also see some metals become cleared from the system as this happens. The theory is that some metals are chelated first and then as they diminish in the body, other metals are then drawn from the tissues and excreted. It's as if the body releases some metals first and then moves on to other metals. This is theory, of course, but it does seem to happen in some patients.

In patients who have mercury-containing dental amalgams, we will always see elevated mercury on the challenge test. It is important to understand that these amalgams do not have a blood supply so whatever is being drawn out does not come directly from the amalgams. The mercury vapors from the amalgams are absorbed in the mucous membranes of the mouth and are also inhaled. Chelating mercury out of someone with amalgams is safe and effective but you will see high mercury levels a year after the detox program due to reaccumulation of mercury from the amalgams. It is best to have them taken out and then commence chelation.

A specific toxic metal detox program goes beyond the scope of this book as there are so many different ways to rid the body of the metals. Since toxic metals can disrupt the function of the thyroid as well as metabolism, it is important to have a basic understanding of where you get them, the symptoms they cause and how to find out if you have them. In my practice, the evaluation of toxic metals tends to be the last resort after we have exhausted all other treatment options. This is due to the fact that most patients get well without addressing toxic metals from the beginning. It is also important to understand that everyone will have some metals come back elevated in the urine challenge test. We all have toxic metals in our systems – especially lead and mercury due to the content of these metals in automobile exhaust and in our air from industry and fossil fuel-burning such as coal. They may cause symptoms in some of us and in others, no problems at all. Make sure you work with someone who understands this and does not think that everyone should be chelated of metals. There are many doctors in practice who think that toxic metals are the cause of almost every health problem and no matter what you come in with, they will treat you for having toxic metals. Each one of you is unique and your diagnosis and treatment plan should reflect your individuality.

CHAPTER NINE
Iodine

Iodine was discovered in 1811 by the French chemist Bernard Courtois. Iodine is an essential element for not only the thyroid but for other body tissues as well. The breast actually requires a fair amount of iodine to be healthy, and women with fibrocystic breast disease have been shown to have low iodine status. In order for iodine to enter the thyroid gland, you must have a healthy transport mechanism which is optimized with vitamin C and magnesium. Twenty-five percent of the iodine in the body is stored in the thyroid gland.

Approximately one-third of the world's population lives in iodine-deficient areas which can lead to thyroid dysfunction and enlargement of the thyroid known as goiter. The recommended daily intake of iodine in North America is 150 micrograms. During pregnancy, the dose is increased to 175 micrograms and then 200 micrograms when breastfeeding. These recommendations were based on preventing goiters but not on optimal thyroid function and the synthesis of T4 and T3. Iodine was added to flour in the 1960s which provided a small dose of iodine per slice of bread. Iodine was replaced by the toxic compound bromide in the early 1980s due to misinformation from the medical community. Bromide is a goitrogen which inhibits the uptake of iodine into the thyroid gland.

Thyroid nodules can form due to an iodine deficiency. Over 95 percent of thyroid nodules are benign and most people will develop a nodule by the time they are fifty. Iodine supplementation has been shown to reduce the size of thyroid nodules. A nuclear thyroid scan can be done to assess if the nodules are "hot" or "cold." Cold nodules should be more thoroughly evaluated as they are the most common type of nodule that are cancerous.

Hypothyroidism and goiter (enlarged thyroid) can result from an iodine deficiency. If the hypothyroidism is congenital, it can lead to mental retardation, lower IQ and stunted growth. The symptoms of iodine deficiency closely relate to those of hypothyroidism which include: weight gain, tenderness around the breast bone, fatigue, cold hands and feet, insomnia, dry eyes, and cracking heels. Iodine was added to table salt to reduce the incidence of goiter but due to recent recommendations to avoid salt, the benefits of iodized salt-reducing goiters has not been maximized. This has led to nearly 200 million Americans with goiters.

Iodine can be found in kelp, seaweed, asparagus, Swiss chard, spinach, seafood and iodized salt. It is important to understand that iodine does not remain in the body for long periods of time so it must be consumed on a regular basis.

Iodine is important not only for the thyroid but also for the prostate gland and breast. Studies have shown that if rats are given iodine-blocking agents, they develop fibrocystic breast disease and calcification. Researchers have also been able to increase breast cancer rates in the animals simply by restricting their intake of iodine. Iodine protects the breast cells from turning cancerous due to its effect on estrogen molecules. Iodine has a similar effect on the prostate gland as well.

A few medical physicians are purported to treat not only thyroid disorders but fibrocystic breast disease, fibromyalgia, chronic fatigue, prostate health and immune function with high doses of iodine. The information that these physicians present is very intriguing but it appears that their original conclusions have gaping holes that must be accounted for. These physicians are promoting high doses of iodine in the range of 12.5-50.0 mg of iodine per day. This is based on research of the average daily intake of Japanese mainlanders. Unfortunately, the studies were misquoted thereby leaving no sound research to support such high doses of iodine. I would like to thank Dr. Jeff Moss of www.mossnutrition.com for his exhaustive research on this topic. If you are a health care practitioner, please visit Dr. Moss's website and read the entire newsletter series on iodine which is the most exhaustive compendium ever compiled on iodine. It will help clarify how much iodine one should take, how much iodine is ingested by the Japanese, its potential negative side effects, and how to test for iodine deficiency.

According to papers published by Aceves and Cann, the average daily dose of iodine intake by Japanese is 5,280 micrograms/day or 5.28 mg/day.[22,23] Also, an FAO/WHO world report states that the average daily intake of iodine by the Japanese is in the range of two to three milligrams per day.[24] Nagataki states in a recent paper: "The average of dietary iodine intake due to the ingestion of seaweeds is 1.2 mg/day in Japan."[25] Contrary to what some medical physicians have led us to believe, experts in Japan do agree that iodine in excess can be detrimental and the average daily dose of 12 mg of iodine per day is false.

What Form of Iodine is Best?

Iodine and iodide have different effects in the body as each one has high affinities for certain glands. Let's clarify these points. Iodide is the most effective form of iodine for the thyroid gland itself. Molecular iodine is the most effective form of iodine for optimal breast health and for the treatment of fibrocystic breasts. We use a product that is a combination of iodine and iodide which contains 1.8 mg per drop. Iodine status can be measured by performing a 24-hour urine collection. This test is done without taking any iodine as some practitioners are promoting. This is an accurate test unlike the iodine patch test. Painting iodine on the skin and recording how long it takes for the stain to go away has no validity whatsoever for iodine status.

The Halides

The halides are a group of elements on the periodic table which interact inside of the body. They include bromine, fluorine, chlorine and iodine. Iodine is a vital nutrient for the health of the thyroid gland but the other halides can negatively affect thyroid function.

Bromide

Bromine is found in kelp/seaweed, nuts, citrus-flavored soft drinks, water purification, pesticides, fumigants, photographic film, dyes, flame retardants, carpet, upholstery, electronics, mattresses and over-the-counter antitussives. Symptoms of bromine toxicity include: gastrointestinal inflammation, asthma, thyroid dysfunction, goiter (enlarged thyroid), headaches, kidney inflammation, low blood pressure and throat inflammation.

Fluoride

Fluorine, also known as fluoride, is found in toothpaste, fluoridated drinking water, infant formula, cereals, non-organic grape juice, wine, beer, soda, tea (higher in decaf), freon, insecticides, fluoridated salt and non-stick coatings. It is also found in many prescription drugs such as anesthetics (Enflurance, Isoflurance, Sevoflurance), fluconazole, fluoroquinolone, antibiotics, Prozac, efavirenz, fluorouracil, flurbiprofen, fenfluramine, cerivastatin, Paxil, fluvoxamine, astemizole, cisapride, fluvastatin, fluocinonide, fluocinolone (topical corticosteroids, fluticasone, flunisolide, fluocinolone acetonide, fludarabine, fludrocortisones) and antimalarial drugs.

Symptoms of fluoride toxicity include: low blood calcium, ligament calcification, bone softening, heart arrhythmias, headaches, nerve pain, vertigo, anemia, lung irritation and male reproductive system toxicity.

Factors That Affect the Uptake of Iodine

Certain drugs can influence the uptake of iodide into the thyroid gland. These include: hydrocortisone, lithium, dexamethasone, sex steroids, RU486, amiodarone, bromide and ketoconazole. Retinoic acid and adenosine actually increase the uptake of iodide into the thyroid.

Foods such as goitrogens can also impact iodine uptake. A goitrogen is a substance that inhibits the uptake of iodide into the thyroid. The goitrogenic activity of a food can be eliminated by lightly cooking, steaming or fermenting. Goitrogens include:

Cassava
Soybeans *(and soybean products such as tofu, soybean oil, soy flour, soy lecithin)*
Pine nuts
Peanuts
Millet
Strawberries

Pears
Peaches
Spinach
Bamboo shoots
Sweet potatoes
Vegetables in the genus Brassica
  Bok choy
  Broccoli
  Broccolini (Asparations)
  Brussels sprouts
  Cabbage
  Canola
  Cauliflower
  Chinese cabbage
  Choy sum
  Collard greens
  Horseradish
  Kai-lan (Chinese broccoli)
  Kale
  Kohlrabi
  Mizuna
  Mustard greens
  Radishes
  Rapeseed (Yu choy)
  Rapini
  Rutabagas
  Tatsoi
  Turnips

What to Consider Before Beginning Iodine Supplementation
With this information in mind, it's clear that iodine can be used safely and effectively but more importantly is the optimization of

iodine flow into and out of the thyroid gland. Too much or too little can significantly affect thyroid function, so how can each person be thoroughly evaluated before commencing iodine supplementation? Finding a functional medicine practitioner such as myself to address these questions is vital. Dr. Jeff Moss presents excellent criteria:

1. Check for genetic predisposition towards thyroid disorders and/ or reactions to iodine supplementation. The best way to clinically determine genetic predisposition is to learn about family history.
2. Evaluate for the presence of systemic inflammation that could adversely affect NIS (iodine transporter) activity using modalities such as clinical examination, white cell count, differential, and C-reactive protein. If present, use functional medicine modalities to reduce inflammation as much as possible.
3. Evaluate for the presence of metal or chemical toxicity. In particular, gain information about the following:

> **Bromide intake**
> **Perchlorate exposure**
> **Tobacco use** *(a significant source of thiocyanate)*
> **Significant intake of natural sources of thiocyanates** *such as vegetables in the brassica family and foods such as cassava, lima beans, linseed, bamboo shoots, and sweet potatoes.*
> **Alcohol use**
> **Commonly used pharmaceuticals** *such as cortisone, testosterone, estrogen, and lithium.*

Key Points About Iodine
The following are the most important points that should be understood about iodine:

1. Iodine is not suitable for every individual.

2. The dose of iodine can be variable for each individual.

3. If you have autoimmune thyroiditis such as Hashimoto's or Graves' disease, you should by no means ever take iodine unless you are under the care of a qualified healthcare practitioner.*

4. Iodine deficiency is a major global issue that needs to be addressed.

5. Many studies have shown that when iodine is added to the food supply to reduce iodine deficiency, the rate of autoimmune thyroiditis increases. Therefore, there is a risk in triggering autoimmunity if you supplement with iodine.

6. Iodine can help treat hypothyroidism and fibrocystic breasts.

7. Iodine improves estrogen metabolism, reduces the risk of developing breast cancer and may do the same for the prostate gland.

*There are too many variables with autoimmune thyroid disease that must be thoroughly evaluated before beginning iodine supplementation due to the fact that iodine can make this condition much worse. Iodine suppresses antibody production giving the illusion that the condition is improving.

CHAPTER TEN
The Thyroid Diet

If you have a thyroid problem, the way you should eat is very similar to that of an individual who does not have a thyroid issue. Organic foods contain fewer amounts of chemicals and pesticides which, as you know from the thyroid-disrupting chemical chapter, can have a negative effect on the thyroid gland. The main goals of a thyroid diet are those which remove any stress from the thyroid gland itself and any systems that may be affecting the thyroid gland. The first major priority in eating to have a healthy thyroid is to make sure you do not have blood sugar swings. This requires consistent eating throughout the day of high-quality protein at every meal without eating too many carbohydrates. Remember that blood sugar swings not only affect the thyroid gland itself but also indirectly affect adrenal gland function which, as previously discussed, is highly connected to thyroid physiology. The ideal protein/carbohydrate intake for someone with thyroid gland dysfunction is to eat a moderate- to low-carbohydrate diet with the exception of post-exercise carbohydrate consumption. The food you consume after you exercise and the meal following your post-workout meal can contain more carbohydrates than you would normally eat. You can do this because your body is much better at handling carbohydrates and blood sugar after you have participated in exercise.

The next important step in optimizing thyroid function is to alkalize your body. Your body contains approximately sixty trillion cells which are involved in six trillion chemical reactions every second. Your cells work best to carry out these chemical processes in an alkaline environment versus an acidic environment. The machinery in your cells that produce energy and burn fat can most easily do their job when the pH is alkaline. Eating foods that drive you into an acidic environment will put undue stress on your cells leading to sub-optimal energy production and function. The best way to find out if you are in an acid or alkaline state is to do a first morning pH test with Hydrion pH strip paper. You should be aiming for a pH of 6.5-7.5. A pH below 6.5 indicates an acidic cellular environment that could be contributing to a decrease in your metabolism. At the same time, you should not be too alkaline which would be a pH above 7.5. This would indicate a catabolic state meaning your body is breaking down its tissues rapidly due to some kind of metabolic or chemical stress. Start by taking your first morning urine pH for five days consecutively. Eliminate the highest and the lowest of the five readings and then average the middle three to attain your pH.

So how do you become more alkaline? The first thing you must do is eat a vegetable or fruit or both at every meal. Produce contains alkaline-forming substances including calcium, magnesium, potassium and zinc. These are "buffering" agents meaning they help to reduce acid by-products of metabolism. The way foods are designated as acid or alkaline is based on the "ash" that is left over when they are burned: the more buffering minerals in the ash, the more alkaline the food. In addition, the protein content of a food will also determine its acid/alkaline status. The presence of more amino acids (protein) in a food leads to more acidity in the body due to amino acid metabolism in the liver resulting in acidic by-products.

Adding sweet potatoes and yams as well as lentils will enhance your alkalinity. In addition, try to eat at least two cups of alkalinizing greens such as kale, mustard greens, turnip greens, or collard greens each day. Lean towards the three most alkalinizing grains: oats (gluten-free if you have Hashimoto's or Graves'), quinoa and wild rice.

There are many other strategies you can use to become more alkaline. Taking an alkalizing bath of one-cup epsom salts and a half-cup of baking soda will aid in alkalizing your body. The epsom salts contain magnesium which is a buffering mineral that will assist in the elimination of acid residues that result from metabolism and detoxification. The baking soda is also extremely alkaline and will aid in neutralizing acidic compounds that the skin is eliminating. Take one of these baths every day, and if you are an athlete, take one at the end of your training day to enhance healing of acidic muscle tissue that has been broken down.

The next thing you can do to alkalize is to drink a morning cocktail of a quarter- to half-teaspoon of unrefined Celtic sea salt, a juiced half-lemon or lime, a greens supplement and a half-teaspoon of buffered vitamin C powder. This cocktail will flood your system with alkalizing agents that mop up acid residues in the body. Please be sure to use unrefined Celtic sea salt which is extremely alkaline as opposed to table salt or sodium chloride which is extremely acidic. Table salt has been stripped of its alkaline minerals resulting in a toxic and acidic product.

Your evening ritual should consist of taking 200 mg of potassium bicarbonate and 100 mg of magnesium glycinate before bed. Increase by one of each until you achieve an alkaline first morning urinary pH.

Acids and bases in the body are also controlled by your breath. Each time you inhale fresh oxygen into the system, your body is preparing to exhale carbon dioxide which, if too high, creates an acidic environment in the blood. Many people in this society are hyperventilators, not taking in full breaths of oxygen and fully exhaling carbon dioxide. The way to remedy this is to engage in deep-belly breathing for five minutes in the morning and five minutes at night. Breathe deeply into the abdomen as if filling your stomach with air and then passively exhale the air without effort. This is how a baby breathes. Concentrate on your breath without thinking about anything else. In time, this will become second nature and you will enjoy doing this twice a day. You can also incorporate this into your meditation practice which you may already be doing. Those of you who do not meditate will reap some of the benefits of meditation as this is a great starting point to learning how to meditate. Focusing on your breathing will focus your thought only on this one task instead of the multitude of things that you think about.

In addition to buffered vitamin C powder, there are a few supplements that can aid in alkalizing the body. Magnesium, potassium bicarbonate, calcium, zinc, fish oil, probiotics and virtually all medicinal herbs will have an alkalizing effect. Herbs and spices that you use for cooking such as turmeric, thyme, oregano, etc. all help to alkalize. In general, meat, dairy and grains are acidic but fruits and vegetables are alkaline. Remember that it is extremely important to eat protein at every meal so do not underconsume protein in fear of becoming too acidic. As long as you are eating vegetables and fruits with each meal, you will become more alkaline. Use the other strategies I have outlined to enhance this process. You will notice many health benefits as you become more alkaline such as an improved sense of well-being, increased energy, fat loss, improved sleep, clearer/sharper mind, improved digestion and a reduction in allergies. Your pH is a sign of your alkaline mineral reserves so be patient in this process. You didn't become acidic overnight so it will take time to reverse an acidic state. It may take you a few months to reach a consistent alkaline state.

How Much Protein Should You Consume?

In addition to developing an alkaline pH, adequate protein intake is a major fundamental aspect of achieving optimal thyroid health. According to the vast majority of nutrition textbooks, healthy individuals should ingest a minimum of 0.8 g of protein per kilogram body weight every day.

Unfortunately, this calculation is not accurate for everyone, because we all have different activity levels, stress levels, and genetics. Another flaw in this calculation is that some of the scientific literature shows that one must ingest 1.2-1.8 g of protein per kilogram body weight every day if there is a protein deficit. Therefore, on average, I prefer for those who are chronically ill to consume 1.2 g of protein per kilogram body weight every day as a minimum. The one exception to this rule is the patient who is producing high amounts of C-reactive protein which is a marker of inflammation. Eating protein will further feed its production by the liver possibly exacerbating your condition.

Another important factor in these calculations is the quality of protein. Not all protein is created equal. So, the amount of protein consumed is heavily dependent on protein sources. Sometimes it can be difficult to get adequate protein intake from diet alone. This is where protein and amino acid supplements come into the picture. Before beginning any kind of protein supplementation, you should be sure that you are eating the highest-quality protein from food sources. These include:

> **Eggs** *(ideally organic and free range)*
> **Types of fish known to be relatively low in heavy metals.**
> **Chicken** *(ideally organic and free range)*
> **Non-commercial forms of red meats such as grass fed, locally raised beef; grass fed buffalo; and grass fed lamb.**
> **Dairy products** *(ideally organic from locally raised dairy cows)*
> **Nuts and seeds, particularly almonds, pecans and walnuts** *(ideally organic)*
> **Legumes** *(ideally organic)*
> **Soybeans**

Since soy allergies are very common, this may be one of the foods on the list that you will need to avoid. In addition, soy products tend to be highly processed. Only soy products that are fermented such as tempeh and miso should be consumed as protein sources from soy.

Dairy is also problematic because of the high allergenicity, processing, and reliability of sources. Dairy can also be very hard to digest and is often contaminated with antibiotics, hormones and toxins from the cows. Dairy is of course an excellent source of protein, but I recommend that the amount of protein consumed from dairy should be minimal.

People are most willing to follow a dietary plan when there are a variety of food choices. This is why I recommend both animal and vegetable-based protein sources eaten in rotation.

Vegan diets can also be a concern regarding protein for a few reasons. If we review the primary protein source of a typical vegan diet in the United States, it is found that soy is the main protein source. Unfortunately, soy is low in sulfur-based amino acids. This is important, because sulfur-based amino acids are required for optimal

liver detoxification, the building of glutathione (a powerful antioxidant) and tissue repair. In addition, plant-based foods contain virtually all of the nutrients necessary for optimal health with the exception of vitamin B12. I find that many, many patients are deficient in B12 and therefore require supplementation. Vegans must have a tremendous amount of knowledge for proper food-combining and supplementation in order to achieve optimal protein and amino acid intake for a healthy body.

When it comes to protein and amino acid supplementation, there are a variety of healthy choices. I recommend whey protein for those who are not sensitive/allergic to dairy. Rice, pea and hemp protein sources can also provide high quality protein and amino acids. Protein powder products are the most beneficial to those who have good digestive function. For those who have impaired digestive function, I like to use free-form amino acid products for direct delivery of protein building blocks into the system. Some people require HCl or digestive enzymes in order to optimize digestion and absorption of amino acids.

Gluten

If you have been diagnosed with Hashimoto's thyroiditis or Graves' disease, you must avoid gluten indefinitely. One of the ways to test for gluten intolerance is the anti-gliadin antibody test which measures an immune response to gliadin, the main protein portion of gluten. A negative anti-gliadin antibody test in saliva, stool or blood does not rule out gluten intolerance. You can still have gluten intolerance and have false negatives on these tests. If the test is positive in saliva, stool or blood then this is a very strong indicator that you are gluten-intolerant. In most cases, there has to be some damage to the lining of the small intestine for the test to be positive in blood or saliva.

It is very important to understand that traditional medicine only recognizes blood testing or small intestine biopsy as diagnostic of gluten intolerance. Your traditional physician will have you go through a "gluten challenge" diet for four to six weeks and then test your blood to see if the gliadin antibody is elevated. This is the worst possible way of detecting gluten intolerance for two reasons. The first is that if someone is gluten-intolerant and you force her to eat gluten for four to six weeks, you are significantly harming her body. The second reason is that this test can be negative even if the person is gluten-intolerant making this test a poor method of diagnosis.

Your traditional doctor may want to order a biopsy of the small intestine to look for damage to the lining of the small intestine. He is looking for what is known as "villous atrophy" meaning the villi that line the gut have been damaged and are worn away from the immune system attack on the dietary gluten intake. The problem with this test is that you can have gluten intolerance but not have villous atrophy. Seventy percent of the negative effects of gluten occur outside of the intestine. This can result in only mild inflammation of the intestine but extra-intestinal damage to organs such as the thyroid, bones, pancreas, brain, adrenals, etc. I would not feel comfortable having a piece of my small intestine cut out just to perform a test that is not completely accurate.

The best thing you can do is to fill out our gluten questionnaire and have the blood, saliva or stool test done to see if there is a positive antibody in any of these. If only one is positive and you have many of the indicators of gluten-intolerance, then you should avoid gluten indefinitely. Most people avoid gluten for a few months and then sneak something in such as a piece of bread and they end up feeling horrible after eating it. Remember – it is estimated that up to 40 percent of Americans are gluten-intolerant so it is very important to know if you are as well. It can mean the difference between a major autoimmune attack on your thyroid or none at all.

The following grains contain gluten:

Wheat
Oats *(not in nature but 99 percent of oats in the US are processed in machinery used for other gluten-containing grains)*
Rye
Barley
Spelt
Kamut
Triticale
Bulgar
Semolina
Couscous
Durum flour

*Gluten can be hidden, so read labels carefully. Be wary of modified food starch, dextrin, flavorings and extracts, hydrolyzed vegetable protein, imitation seafood, and creamed or thickened products such as soups, stews, and sauces.

The following grains do not contain gluten and are acceptable for gluten-intolerant individuals and of course those who are not:

Corn
Millet
Rice
Taro
Teff
Arrowroot
Wild Rice
Tapioca
Buckwheat
Quinoa
Amaranth
Wheat Grass
Barley Grass
Barley Malt

Goitrogens

Goitrogens are compounds in certain foods that inhibit the uptake of iodine into the thyroid gland. Goitrogens can be neutralized by lightly steaming, fermenting or cooking these foods. Foods that contain goitrogens include: kale, cabbage, turnips, rape seeds, peanuts, cassava, sweet potatoes, soybeans, kelp and Brassica vegetables such as broccoli and brussels sprouts. All of these foods eaten in their raw state could have goitrogenic activity on the thyroid gland.

Final Thoughts

I hope that this book has made you understand that there can be many causes to your thyroid problem. It takes a skilled functional medicine physician to find the underlying cause of your thyroid problem and teach you how to correct it permanently. In rare cases, you may have to take thyroid hormone but going through the processes outlined in this book will help your thyroid work so much better if you do need medication. I do not believe that 27 million Americans were born with defective thyroid glands. It is the combination of environmental stresses, imbalanced systems of the body, nutritional deficiencies, autoimmunity, etc. that lead to thyroid symptoms and imbalances. Once all of these causative factors are identified and corrected, the thyroid gland can function optimally and you can regain the vibrant health that you once had.

We are coming to the end of the dark ages of medicine. The days of identifying symptoms, myopically looking at single lab tests and then prescribing a toxic drug to mask symptoms will soon be over. We now have the technology and the understanding of human physiology to significantly turn someone's life around and help the individual achieve recovery from illness.

This book has provided you with a concise and clear understanding of all of the possible causes of thyroid dysfunction. As you can see, it's not just a matter of taking a pill to fix your thyroid problem. You can certainly choose to do this but for those of you who really want to get to the underlying cause of your thyroid problem, you must work with someone who understands the concepts outlined in this book. I have successfully worked with patients all over the United States and even in other countries from a distance. Fortunately, I am able to order lab tests anywhere in the United States and I converse with patients via telephone and Internet video chat. We are able to consult and cover all of your lab tests and implement treatment plans from afar. I can also work closely with your physician as a team to get you well. Please contact me with any questions or concerns about your case which I am happy to review.

Yours in Health,
Dr. Nikolas R. Hedberg

Resources

Dr. Hedberg's office:
Functional Diagnostic Medical Center
141 Asheland Ave. Suite 301
Asheville, NC 28801
Phone: 828-254-4024
www.drhedberg.com
info@drhedberg.com
Facebook: www.facebook.com/DrNikolasHedberg
Twitter: www.twitter.com/drhedberg

Supplement Companies Dr. Hedberg Utilizes:
Moss Nutrition
800-851-5444
www.mossnutrition.com
Moss Nutrition distributes the top supplement companies Dr. Hedberg utilizes including Klaire Labs & Designs for Health

Laboratories Recommended by Dr. Hedberg:
Metametrix Clinical Laboratory
3425 Corporate Way
Duluth, GA 30096
www.metametrix.com
Phone: 800-221-4640
Utilized Tests: GIFx stool test, Organic acids, Porphyrins, Amino Acids, Fatty Acids, Adrenal Stress ,
Toxic Metal & Chemical Profiles, Designs For Health Metabolic Profiles

LabCorp
www.labcorp.com
Utilized Tests: Conventional blood chemistries including thyroid, cholesterol, metabolic profiles etc.

Professional Co-op Services
www.professionalco-op.com
Phone: 866-999-4041
Utilized Tests: Provides all LabCorp tests at a discounted price
for cash patients.

Where to find a mercury-free dentist:
www.iaomt.org

Environmental Toxin Resource:
Environmental Working Group
www.ewg.org
Utilize their cosmetic database for thyroid disrupting chemicals

References

1.   Baker SM, Bennett P, Bland JS, et al. *The Textbook of Functional Medicine*. Gig Harbor, WA: Institute for Functional Medicine; 2005.

2.   Baker SM, Bennett P, Bland JS, et al. *The Textbook of Functional Medicine*. Gig Harbor, WA: Institute for Functional Medicine; 2005.

3.   Baker SM, Bennett P, Bland JS, et al. *The Textbook of Functional Medicine*. Gig Harbor, WA: Institute for Functional Medicine; 2005.

4.   Baker SM, Bennett P, Bland JS, et al. *The Textbook of Functional Medicine*. Gig Harbor, WA: Institute for Functional Medicine; 2005.

5.   Baker SM, Bennett P, Bland JS, et al. *The Textbook of Functional Medicine*. Gig Harbor, WA: Institute for Functional Medicine; 2005.

6.   Obál F Jr., Krueger JM. The somatotropic axis and sleep. *Rev Neurol*. 2001 Nov;157,(11 Pt 2):S12-5. Review.

7.   Benvenga S, Amato A, Calvani M, Trimarchi F. Effects of Carnitine on Thyroid Hormone Action from Carnitine: The Science Behind a Conditionally Essential Nutrient. *Annals of the New York Academy of Sciences*. Nov 2004;Vol 1033:ix-xi,1-197.

8.   Tomer Y, Davies TF. Infection, thyroid disease, and autoimmunity. *Endocr Rev*. 1993 Feb;14(1):107-20. Review.

9.   Valentino R et al. Prevalence of coeliac disease in patients with thyroid autoimmunity. *Horm Res*. 1999;51(3):124-27.

10.   Sterzl I et al. Removal of dental amalgam decreases anti-TPO and anti-Tg autoantibodies in patients with autoimmune thyroiditis. *Neuro Endocrinol Lett*. 2006 Dec;27 Suppl 1:25-30. Erratum in: *Neuro Endocrinol Lett*. 2007 Oct;28(5):iii.

11.   Braverman MD, LE, Utiger MD, RD. Werner and Ingbar's The *Thyroid: A Fundamental and Clinical Text*. Philadelphia, PA: Lippincott Williams & Wilkins; 2000.

12.   EPA website: www.epa.gov/epahome/resource.htm. August 2009.

13.   EPA website: www.epa.gov/epahome/resource.htm. August 2009.

14.   EPA website: www.epa.gov/epahome/resource.htm. August 2009.

15. Zoeller RT, 2007 Environmental chemicals impacting the thyroid: Targets and consequences. *Thyroid*. 2007;17:811-17.

16. Zoeller RT, 2007 Environmental chemicals impacting the thyroid: Targets and consequences. *Thyroid*. 2007;17:811-17.

17. Zoeller RT et al. Developmental exposure to polychlorinated biphenyls exerts thyroid hormone-like effects on the expression of RC3/neurogranin and myelin basic protein messenger ribonucleic acids in the developing rat brain. *Endocrinology*. 2000;141:181-89.

18. Zoeller RT. *Polychlorinated biphenyls as disruptors of thyroid hormone action*. In Fisher LJ, Hansen L , editors. PCBs: *Recent advances in the environmental toxicology and health effects of PCBs*. Lexington: University of Kentucky Press; 265-72.

19. Tan SW et al. The endocrine effects of mercury in humans and wildlife. *Crit Rev Toxicol*. 2009;39(3):228-69. Review.

20. Kawada J et al. Effects of organic and inorganic mercurials on thyroidal functions. *J Pharmacobiodyn*. 1980 Mar;3(3):149-59.

21. Aceves C et al. Is iodine a gatekeeper of the integrity of the mammary gland? *J Mammary Gland Biol Neoplasia*. 2005;10(2):189-96.

22. Cann SA et al. Hypothesis: iodine, selenium and the development of breast cancer. *Cancer Causes Control*. 2000;11(2):121-7.

23. Moss, J DDS. (2007). A Perspective on High Dose Iodine Supplementation-Part V-The Japanese Experiment with Dietary Iodine. *Moss Nutrition Report* #218.

24. Nagataki S. The average of dietary iodine intake due to the ingestion of seaweeds is 1.2 mg/day in Japan. *Thyroid*. 2008;18(6):667-68.

25. Aakvaag A, Sand T, Opstad PK, Fonnum F. Hormonal changes in serum in young men during prolonged physical strain. *Eur J Appl Physiol Occup Physiol*. 1978 Oct; 20;39(4):283-91.

26. Niepomniszcze H, Pitoia F, Katz SB, Chervin R, Bruno OD. Primary thyroid disorders in endogenous Cushing's syndrome. *Eur J Endocrinol*. 2002 Sep;147(3):305-11.

27. Surks MI, et al. Subclinical thyroid disease: Scientific review and guidelines for diagnosis and management. *JAMA*. 2004;291(2): 228-238.

28. American College of Obstetricians and Gynecologists Thyroid Disease in Pregnancy. ACOG Practice Bulletin No. 37. *Obstetrics and Gynecology.* 2002;100(2): 387–396.

29. Berkow R, Fletcher AJ (eds.) *The Merck Manual*, edition 16. Rahway, NJ: Merck & Co.; 1992.

30. Guyton AC, Hall JE. *Textbook of Medical Physiology*, edition 9. Philadelphia, PA: W. B. Saunders; 1996.

31. Schaff L, et al. Screening for thyroid disorders in a working population. *Clin Investig.* 1993;71:126-31.

32. Helfand M, Crapo L. Screening for thyroid disease, *Ann Intern Med.* 1990;112:840-9.

33. Rallison, et al. Natural history of thyroid abnormalities: prevalence, incidence, and regression of thyroid disease in adolescents and young adults. *Am J Med.* 1991;91363-9.

34. Fischbach F. *A Manual of Laboratory & Diagnostic Tests*, 5th edition. Philadelphia, PA: J. B. Lippincott Co.; 1996.

35. Costa AJ. Interpreting thyroid tests. *Am Fam Physician.* 1995;52(8):2325-30.

36. The Broda Barnes, M.D. Research Foundation, Inc. P.O. Box 98, Trumble, CT 06611.

37. Werbach MR. *Nutritional Influences on Illness*, edition 2. Tarzana: Third Line Press; 1996.

38. Williamson M. Thyroid dysfunction and its somatic reflection: a preliminary report. *J Am Osteopath Assoc.* 1973;72:105-11.

39. Barnes BO. *Hypothyroidism: The Unsuspected Illness*. New York, NY: Harper & Row; 1976.

40. Auf'mkolk M, Ingbar JC, Kubota K, et al. Extracts and auto-oxidized constituents of certain plants inhibit the receptor-binding and biological activity of Graves' immunoglobulins. *Endocrin.*1985;116:1687-93.

41. Brinker, F. Inhibition of Endocrine Function by Botanical Agents. *J Naturopathic Medicine.* v. 1 number 1.

42. Wagner H, Horhammer L, Frank U. Lithospermic acid, the anti-

hormonally active principle of Lycopus europaeus L. and Symphytum officinale L., *Arzneim Forsch*. 1970; 20:705-12.

43.   Winterhoff H, Gumbinger HG, Vahlensieck U, et al. Endocrine effects of Lycopus europaeus L. following oral application. *Arzneimittl-forschung*. 1994;44:41-5.

44.   Blumenthal M, Busse WR, Goldberg A, et al. (eds). *The Complete Commission E Monographs: Therapeutic Guide to Herbal Medicines*. Boston, MA: Integrative Medicine Communications; 1998:98-9.

45.   Beard JL, Borel MJ, Derr J. Impaired thermoregulation and thyroid function in iron-deficiency anemia, *Am J Clin Nutr*. 1990 Nov;52(5):813-9.

46.   Köhrle J. The deiodinase family: selenoenzymes regulating thyroid hormone availability and action. *Cell Mol Life Sci*. 2000 Dec; 57(13-14):1853-63. Review.

47.   Berry MJ, Larsen PR.The role of selenium in thyroid hormone action. *Endocr Rev*. 1992 May;13(2):207-19. Review.

48.   Brzezińska-Slebodzińska E. Fever induced oxidative stress: the effect on thyroid status and the 5'-monodeiodinase activity, protective role of selenium and vitamin E. *J Physiol Pharmacol*. 2001 Jun;52(2):275-84.

49.   Duntas LH. The role of selenium in thyroid autoimmunity and cancer. *Thyroid*. 2006 May;16(5):455-60.

50.   Nishiyama S, Nishiyama S, Futagoishi-Suginohara Y, Matsukura M, Nakamura T, Higashi A, Shinohara M, Matsuda I. Zinc supplementation alters thyroid hormone metabolism in disabled patients with zinc deficiency. *J Am Coll Nutr*. 1994 Feb; 13(1):62-7.

51.   Pansini F, Bassi P, Cavallini AR, Ambrosecchia R, Bergamini CM, Meduri P, Bagni B. Effect of the hormonal contraception on serum reverse triiodothyronine levels. *Gynecol Obstet Invest*. 1987; 23(2):133-4.

52.   Doerge DR, Chang HC. Inactivation of thyroid peroxidase by soy isoflavones, in vitro and in vivo. *J Chromatogr B Analyt Technol Biomed Life Sci*. 2002 Sep 25;777(1-2):269-79. Review.

53.   Divi RL, Chang HC, Doerge DR. Anti-thyroid isoflavones from soybean: isolation, characterization, and mechanisms of action. *Bio-*

chem Pharmacol. 1997 Nov 15;54(10):1087-96.

54.   Bunevicius R, Kazanavicius G, Zalinkevicius R, Prange AJ Jr. Effects of thyroxine as compared with thyroxine plus triiodothyronine in patients with hypothyroidism. *N Engl J Med*. 1999 Feb 11;340(6):424-9.

55.   Visser TJ. Role of sulfation in thyroid hormone metabolism. *Chem Biol Interact*. 1994 Jun;92(1-3):293-303. Review.

56.   Diamanti-Kandarakis E, Palioura E, Kandarakis SA, Koutsilieris M. Thyroid Disrupting Chemicals: The impact of endocrine disruptors on endocrine targets. *Horm Metab Res*. 2010 Jul;42(8):543-52. Epub 2010 Apr 23. Review.

57.   Decherf S, Seugnet I, Fini JB, Clerget-Froidevaux MS, Demeneix BA. Disruption of thyroid hormone-dependent hypothalamic setpoints by environmental contaminants. *Mol Cell Endocrinol*. 2010 Jul 29;323(2):172-82. Epub 2010 Apr 24.

58.   Zoeller TR. Environmental chemicals targeting thyroid. *Hormones* (Athens). 2010 Jan-Mar;9(1):28-40. Review.

59.   Kelly GS. Peripheral metabolism of thyroid hormones: A review. *Altern Med Rev*. 2000;5:306-333.

60.   Richardson VM, Staskal DF, Ross DG, Diliberto JJ, DeVito MJ, Birnbaum LS. Possible mechanisms of thyroid hormone disruption in mice by BDE 47, a major polybrominated diphenyl ether congener. *Toxicol Appl Pharmacol*. 2008;226: 244-250.

61.   Zoeller RT. Thyroid toxicology and brain development: Should we think differently? *Environ Health Perspect*. 2003;111: A628.

62.   Brucker-Davis F. Effects of environmental synthetic chemicals on thyroid function. *Thyroid*. 1998;8: 827-856.

63.   Schantz SL, Widholm JJ, Rice DC. Effects of PCB exposure on neuropsychological function in children. *Environ Health Perspect*. 2003;111: 357-576.

64.   Stewart PW, Reihman J, Lonky EI, Darvill TJ, Pagano J. Cognitive development in preschool children prenatally exposed to PCBs and MEHG. *Neurotoxicol Teratol*. 2003; 25:11-22.

65.   Stewart PW, Lonky E, Reihman J, Pagano J, Gump BB, Darvill T. The relationship between prenatal PCB exposure and intelligence (IQ)

in 9-year-old children. *Environ Health Perspect.* 2008;116:1416-1422.

66. Bastomsky CH. Enhanced thyroxine metabolism and high uptake goiters in rats after a single dose of 2,3,7,8-tetrachlorodibenzo-p-dioxin. *Endocrinol.* 1998;101:292-296.

67. Gauger KJ, Sharlin DS, Zoeller RT (eds.). Polychlorinated biphenyls as disruptors of thyroid hormone action. In: ed. Champagne-Urbana, University of Illinois Press. (2007).

68. Zoeller RT. Polychlorinated biphenyls as disruptors of thyroid hormone action. In Fisher LJ, Hansen L (eds): *PCBs: Recent advances in the environmental toxicology and health effects of PCBs.* Lexington, University of Kentucky Press. (2001). pp.265-272.

69. Murai K, Okamura K, Tsuji H, et al. Thyroid function in "Yusho" Patients exposed to polychlorinated biphenyls (PCB). *Environ Res.* 1987; 44:179-187.

70. Goldey ES, Kehn LS, Lau C, Rehnberg GL, Crofton KM. Developmental exposure to polychlorinated biphenyls (aroclor 1254) reduces circulating thyroid hormone concentrations and causes hearing deficits in rats. *Toxicol Appl Pharmacol.* 1995;135:77-88.

71. Salay E, Garabrant D. Polychlorinated biphenyls and thyroid hormones in adults: A systematic review appraisal of epidemiological studies. *Chemosphere.* 2009;74:1413-1419.

72. Herbstman JB, Sjodin A, Apelberg BJ, et al. Birth delivery mode modifies the associations between prenatal polychlorinated biphenyl (PCB) and polybrominated diphenyl ether (PBDE) and neonatal thyroid hormone levels. *Environ Health Perspect.* 2008;116:1376-1382.

73. Zoeller RT, Dowling AL, Vas AA. Developmental exposure to polychlorinated biphenyls exerts thyroid hormone-like effects on the expression of RC3/neurogranin and myelin basic protein messenger ribonucleic acids in the developing rat brain. *Endocrinology.* 2000;141:181-189.

74. Tseng LH, Li MH, Tsai SS, et al. Developmental exposure to decabromodiphenyl ether (PBDE 209): Effects on thyroid hormone and hepatic enzyme activity in male mouse offspring. *Chemosphere.* 2008;70:640-647.

75. Darnerud PO, Aune M, Larsson L, Hallgren S. Plasma PBDE and

thyroxine levels in rats exposed to bromkal or BDE-47. *Chemosphere*. 2007;67:S386-392.

76.   Hallgren S, Sinjari T, Hakansson H, Darnerud PO. Effects of poly-brominated diphenyl ethers (PBDEs) and polychlorinated biphenyls (PCBs) on thyroid hormone and vitamin A levels in rats and mice. *Arch Toxicol*. 2001;75:200-208.

77.   Greer MA, Goodman G, Pleus RC, Greer SE, 2002 Health effects assessment for environmental perchlorate contamination: The dose response for inhibition of thyroidal radioiodine uptake in humans. *Environ Health Perspect*. 2002;110:927-937.

78.   Blount BC, Pirkle JL, Osterloh JD, Valentin-Blasini L, Caldwell KL. Urinary perchlorate and thyroid hormone levels in adolescent and adult men and women living in the United States. *Environ Health Perspect*. 2006;114:1865-1871.

79.   Steinmaus C, Miller MD, Howd R. Impact of smoking and thiocyanate on perchlorate and thyroid hormone associations in the 2001-2002 National Health and Nutrition Examination Survey. *Environ Health Perspect*. 2007;115:1333-1338.

80.   Lawrence J, Lamm S, Braverman LE. Low dose perchlorate (3 mg daily) and thyroid function. *Thyroid*. 2001;11:295.

81.   Lawrence JE, Lamm SH, Pino S, Richman K, Braverman LE. The effect of short-term low-dose perchlorate on various aspects of thyroid function. *Thyroid*. 2000;10:659-663.

82.   Moriyama K, Tagami T, Akamizu T, et al. Thyroid hormone action is disrupted by bisphenol-A as an antagonist. *J Clin Endocrinol Metab*. 2002;87:5185-5190.

83.   Jung KK, Kim SY, Kim TG, et al. Differential regulation of thyroid hormone receptor-mediated function by endocrine disruptors. *Arch Pharm Res*. 2007; 30: 616-623

84.   Heimeier RA, Das B, Buchholz DR, Shi YB. The xenoestrogen bisphenol-A inhibits postembryonic vertebrate development by antagonizing gene regulation by thyroid hormone. *Endocrinology*. 2009;150:2964-2973.

85.   Sun H, Shen OX, Wang XR, Zhou L, Zhen SQ, Chen XD. Anti-thyroid hormone activity of bisphenol-A, tetrabromobisphenol-A and

tetrachlorobisphenol-A in an improved reporter gene assay. *Toxicol In Vitro*. 2009;23:950-954.

86. Yen PM. Molecular basis of resistance to thyroid hormone. T*rends Endocrinol Metab*. 2003;14:327-333.

87. Benvenga S, Guarneri F, Vaccaro M, Santarpia L, Trimarchi F. Homologies between proteins of Borrelia burgdorferi and thyroid autoantigens. *Thyroid*. 2004 Nov;14(11):964-6.

88. Hybenova M, Hrda P, Procházková J, Stejskal V, Sterzl I. The role of environmental factors in autoimmune thyroiditis. *Neuro Endocrinol Lett*. 2010;31(3):283-9. Review.

89. Wang J, Zhang W, Liu H, Wang D, Wang W, Li Y, Wang Z, Wang L, Zhang W, Huang G. Parvovirus B19 infection associated with Hashimoto's thyroiditis in adults. *J Infect*. 2010 May;60(5):360-70. Epub 2010 Feb 12.

90. Stechova K, Pomahacova R, Hrabak J, Durilova M, Sykora J, Chudoba D, Stavikova V, Flajsmanova K, Varvarovska J. Reactivity to Helicobacter pylori antigens in patients suffering from thyroid gland autoimmunity. *Exp Clin Endocrinol Diabetes*. 2009 Sep;117(8):423-31. Epub 2009 May 26.

91. Antonelli A, Ferri C, Fallahi P, Ferrari SM, Frascerra S, Pampana A, Panicucci E, Carpi A, Nicolini A, Ferrannini E. CXCL10 and CCL2 chemokine serum levels in patients with hepatitis C associated with autoimmune thyroiditis. *J Interferon Cytokine Res*. 2009 Jun;29(6):345-51

92. Desailloud R, Hober D. Viruses and thyroiditis: an update. *Virol J*. 2009 Jan 12;6:5. Review.

93. Corapçioğlu D, Tonyukuk V, Kiyan M, Yilmaz AE, Emral R, Kamel N, Erdoğan G. Relationship between thyroid autoimmunity and Yersinia enterocolitica antibodies. *Thyroid*. 2002 Jul;12(7):613-7.

94. Chatzipanagiotou S, Legakis JN, Boufidou F, Petroyianni V, Nicolaou C. Prevalence of Yersinia plasmid-encoded outer protein (Yop) class-specific antibodies in patients with Hashimoto's thyroiditis. *Clin Microbiol Infect*. 2001 Mar;7(3):138-43.

95. Kannangai R, Sachithanandham J, Kandathil AJ, Ebenezer DL, Danda D, Vasuki Z, Thomas N, Vasan SK, Sridharan G. Immune responses to Epstein-Barr virus in individuals with systemic and organ

specific autoimmune disorders. *Indian J Med Microbiol*. 2010 Apr-Jun;28(2):120-3.

96. Thomas D, Karachaliou F, Kallergi K, Vlachopapadopoulou E, Antonaki G, Chatzimarkou F, Fotinou A, Kaldrymides P, Michalacos S. Herpes virus antibodies seroprevalence in children with autoimmune thyroid disease. *Endocrine*. 2008 Apr;33(2):171-5. Epub 2008 May 13.

97. Espino Montoro A, Medina Pérez M, González Martín MC, Asencio Marchante R, López Chozas JM. Subacute thyroiditis associated with positive antibodies to the Epstein-Barr virus. *An Med Interna*. 2000 Oct;17(10):546-8. Review.

98. Kawada J, Nishida M, Yoshimura Y, Mitani K. Effects of organic and inorganic mercurials on thyroidal functions. *J Pharmacobiodyn*. 1980 Mar;3(3):149-59.

99. Nishida M, Matsumoto H, Asano A, Umazume K, Yoshimura Y, Kawada J. Direct evidence for the presence of methylmercury bound in the thyroid and other organs obtained from mice given methylmercury; differentiation of free and bound methylmercuries in biological materials determined by volatility of methylmercury. *Chem Pharm Bull*. (Tokyo). 1990 May;38(5):1412-3.

100. Prochazkova J, Sterzl I, Kucerova H, Bartova J, Stejskal VD. The beneficial effect of amalgam replacement on health in patients with autoimmunity. *Neuro Endocrinol Lett*. 2004 Jun;25(3):211-8.

101. Bártová J, Procházková J, Krátká Z, Benetková K, Venclíková Z, Sterzl I. Dental amalgam as one of the risk factors in autoimmune diseases. *Neuro Endocrinol Lett*. 2003 Feb-Apr;24(1-2):65-7.

102. Sterzl I, Procházková J, Hrdá P, Bártová J, Matucha P, Stejskal VD. Mercury and nickel allergy: risk factors in fatigue and autoimmunity. *Neuro Endocrinol Lett*.1999;20(3-4):221-228.

103. Sterzl I, Hrdá P, Procházková J, Bártová J, Matucha P. Reactions to metals in patients with chronic fatigue and autoimmune endocrinopathy. *Vnitr Lek*. 1999 Sep;45(9):527-31. Czech.

104. Vas J, Monestier M. Immunology of mercury. *Ann N Y Acad Sci*. 2008 Nov;1143:240-67. Review.

105. Caride A, Fernández-Pérez B, Cabaleiro T, Tarasco M, Esquifino AI, Lafuente A. Cadmium chronotoxicity at pituitary level: effects on

plasma ACTH, GH, and TSH daily pattern. *J Physiol Biochem.* 2010 Sep;66(3):213-20. Epub 2010 Jul 22.

106. Hammouda F, Messaoudi I, El Hani J, Baati T, Saïd K, Kerkeni A. Reversal of cadmium-induced thyroid dysfunction by selenium, zinc, or their combination in rat. *Biol Trace Elem Res.* 2008 Winter;126(1-3):194-203. Epub 2008 Aug 8.

107. Davey JC, Nomikos AP, Wungjiranirun M, Sherman JR, Ingram L, Batki C, Lariviere JP, Hamilton JW. Arsenic as an endocrine disruptor: arsenic disrupts retinoic acid receptor-and thyroid hormone receptor-mediated gene regulation and thyroid hormone-mediated amphibian tail metamorphosis. *Environ Health Perspect.* 2008 Feb;116(2):165-72.

108. Meltzer HM, Maage A, Ydersbond TA, Haug E, Glattre E, Holm H. Fish arsenic may influence human blood arsenic, selenium, and T4:T3 ratio. *Biol Trace Elem Res.* 2002 Winter;90(1-3):83-98.

109. Akçay MN, Akçay G. The presence of the antigliadin antibodies in autoimmune thyroid diseases. *Hepatogastroenterology.* 2003 Dec;50 Suppl 2:cclxxix-cclxxx.

110. Valentino R, Savastano S, Tommaselli AP, Dorato M, Scarpitta MT, Gigante M, Micillo M, Paparo F, Petrone E, Lombardi G, Troncone R. Prevalence of coeliac disease in patients with thyroid autoimmunity. *Horm Res.* 1999;51(3):124-7.

111. Cuoco L, Certo M, Jorizzo RA, De Vitis I, Tursi A, Papa A, De Marinis L, Fedeli P, Fedeli G, Gasbarrini G. Prevalence and early diagnosis of coeliac disease in autoimmune thyroid disorders. *Ital J Gastroenterol Hepatol.* 1999 May;31(4):283-7.

112. Valentino R, Savastano S, Maglio M, Paparo F, Ferrara F, Dorato M, Lombardi G, Troncone R. Markers of potential coeliac disease in patients with Hashimoto's thyroiditis. *Eur J Endocrinol.* 2002 Apr;146(4):479-83.

113. Miller DW. Extrathyroid benefits of iodine. *J Amer Physicians and Surgeons.* 2006;11(4):106-110.

114. Pearce EN et al. Effects of chronic iodine excess in a cohort of long-term American workers in West Africa. *J Clin Endocrinol Metab.* 2002;87(12):5499-5502.

115. Hollowell J et al. Iodine nutrition in the United States. Trends and

public health implications: Iodine excretion data from national health and nutrition examination surveys I and III (1971-1974 and 1988-1994). *J Clin Endocrinol Metab*. 1998;83:3401-3408.

116. Ghent W et al. Iodine replacement in fibrocystic disease of the breast. *Can J Surg*. 1993;36:453-460.

117. Meletis CD & Zabriskie N. Iodine, a critically overlooked nutrient. *Alternative & Complimentary Therapies*. 2007 June;132-136.

118. Smyth PPA. Role of iodine in antioxidant defence in thyroid and breast disease. *Biofactors*. 2003;1(3-4):121-130.

119. Aceves C et al. Is iodine a gatekeeper of the integrity of the mammary gland? *J Mammary Gland Biol Neoplasia*. 2005;10(2):189-96.

120. Venturi S. Is there a role for iodine in breast diseases? *The Breast*. 2001;10(5):379-82.

121. Cann SA et al. Hypothesis: iodine, selenium and the development of breast cancer. *Cancer Causes Control*. 2000;11(2):121-7.

122. Ghent W et al. Iodine replacement in fibrocystic disease of the breast. *Can J Surg*. 1993;36:453-460.

123. Kessler JH. The effect of supraphysiologic levels of iodine on patients with cyclic mastalgia. *Breast J*. 2004;10(4):328-36.

124. Smyth PP. The thyroid, iodine and breast cancer. *Breast Cancer Res*. 2003;5(5):R110-3.

125. Studies of hypothyroidism in patients with high iodine intake. *J Clin Endocrinol Metab*. 1986;63(2):412-417. Kapil U et al.

126. Nagataki S et al. Benefits and safety of dietary iodine intake in India. *Pakistan J Nutr*. 2003;2(1):43-45.

127. Nagataki S et al. Thyroid function in chronic excess iodide ingestion: Comparison of thyroidal absolute iodine uptake and degradation of thyroxine in euthyroid Japanese subjects. *J Clin Endocrinol Metab*. 1967;27(5):638-647.

128. Konno N et al. Gaby AR. Editorial: Iodine: A lot to swallow. *Townsend Letter for Doctors & Patients*. 2005(August/September 2005).

129. Konno N et al. Association between dietary iodine intake and prevalence of subclinical hypothyroidism in the coastal regions of Japan. *J Clin Endocrinol Metab*. 1994;78(2):393-397.

130. Murakami, S. Screening for thyroid diseases in an iodine sufficient area with sensitive thyrotrophin assays, and serum thyroid autoantibody and urinary iodide determinations (Abstract). *Clin Endocrinol (Oxf)* . 1993;38(3):273-81.

131. Smyth PPA & Dwyer RM. The sodium iodide symporter and thyroid disease. *Clin Endocrinol (Oxf)*. 2002;56:427-429.

132. Saito T et al. Increased expression of the Na+/I- symporter in cultured human thyroid cells exposed to thyrotrophin and in Graves' thyroid tissue. *J Clin Endocrinol Metab*. 1997;82(10):3331-3336.

133. De La Viega A et al. Molecular analysis of the sodium/iodide symporter: Impact on thyroid and extrathyroid pathophysiology. *Physiol Rev*. 2000;80(3):1083-1105.

134. Hou X et al. Determination of chemical species of iodine in some seaweeds. *Science of the Total Environment*. 1997;204(3):215-221.

135. Schroder-van der Elst JP et al. Dietary flavonoids and iodine metabolism. *Biofactors*. 2003;19:171-176.

136. Shen DHY et al. Sodium iodide symporter in health and disease. *Thyroid*. 2001;11(5):415-425.

137. Konno N et al. Association between dietary iodine intake and prevalence of subclinical hypothyroidism in the coastal regions of Japan. *J Clin Endocrinol Metab*. 1994;78(2):393-397.

138. Koutras DA et al. Effect of small iodine supplements on thyroid function in normal individuals. *J Clin Endocrinol*. 1964;24:857-862.

139. Nagataki S et al. Thyroid function in chronic excess iodide ingestion: Comparison of thyroidal absolute iodine uptake and degradation of thyroxine in euthyroid Japanese subjects. *J Clin Endocrinol Metab*. 1967;27(5):638-647.

140. Skare S & Frey HM. Iodine induced thyrotoxicosis in apparently normal thyroid glands. *Acta Endocrinologica (Copenh)*. 1980;94(3):332-6.

141. Zois C et al. Natural course of autoimmune thyroiditis after

elimination of iodine deficiency in northwestern Greece. *Thyroid.* 2006;16(3):289-93.

142. Zois C et al. High prevalence of autoimmune thyroiditis in school-children afater elimination of iodine deficiency in northwestern Greece. *Thyroid.* 2003;13(5):485-9.

143. Bastemir M et al. High prevalence of thyroid dysfunction and auto-immune thyroiditis in adolescents after elimination of iodine deficiency in the Eastern Black Sea Region of Turkey. *Thyroid.* 2006;16(12):1265-71.

144. Pedersen IB et al. An increased incidence of overt hypothyroidism after iodine fortification of salt in Denmark: A prospective population study. *J Clin Endocrinol Metab.* 2007;92:3122-3127.

145. Papanastasiou L et al. Thyroid autoimmunity in the current iodine environment. *Thyroid.* 2007;17(8):729-739.

146. Todd CH & Dunn JT. Intermittent oral administration of potassium iodide solution for the correction of iodine deficiency. *Am J Clin Nutr.* 1998;67:1279-83.

147. Paul T et al. The effect of small increases in dietary iodine on thyroid function in euthyroid subjects. *Metabolism.* 1988;37(2):121-124.

148. Gardner DF et al. Effects of low dose iodide supplementation on thyroid function in normal men. *Clin Endocrinol (Oxf).* 1988;28(3):283-8.

149. Stadel BV. Dietary iodine and risk of breast, endometrial, and ovarian cancer. *Lancet.* 1976;1(7965):890-1.

150. Clur A. Di-iodothyronine as part of the oestradiol and catechol oestrogen receptor -- the role of iodine, thyroid hormones and melatonin in the aetiology of breast cancer. *Med Hypotheses.* 1988;27:303-311.

151. Lord RS et al. Estrogen metabolism and the diet-cancer connection: Rationale for assessing the ratio of urinary hydroxylated estrogen metabolites. *Alt Med Rev.* 2002;7(2):112-129.

152. Stoddard FR et al. Iodine alters gene expression in the MCF7 breast cancer cell line: Evidence for an anti-estrogen effect of iodine. *Int J Med Sci.* 2008;5(4):189-196.

153. Rogan EG et al. Relative imbalances in estrogen metabolism and

conjugation in breast tissue of women with carcinoma: potential bio-markers of susceptibility to cancer. *Carcinogenesis*. 2003;24(4):697-702.

154. Slebodzinski AB. Ovarian iodide uptake and triiodothyronine generation in follicular fluid: The enigma of the thyroid ovary interaction. *Domestic Animal Endocrinology*. 2005;29:97-103.

155. Pavelka S. Metabolism of bromide and its interference with the metabolism of iodine. *Physiol Res*. 2004;53(Suppl 1):S81-S90.

156. Kurokawa Y et al. Toxicity and carcinogenicity of potassium bromate - A new renal carcinogen. *Environ Health Perspectives*. 1990;87:309-335.

157. van Leeuwen FX et al. Toxicity of sodium bromide in rats: effects on endocrine system and reproduction. *Food Chem Toxicol*. 1983;21(4):383-9.

158. Vobecky M & Babicky A. Effect of enhanced bromide intake on the concentration ratio I/Br in the rat thyroid gland. *Biol Trace Elem Res*. 1994;43-45(Fall):509-16.

159. Velicky J et al. Potassium bromide and the thyroid gland of the rat: morphology and immunochemistry, RIA and INAA analysis. *Ann Anat*. 1997;179(5):421-31.

160. Sangster B et al. The influence of sodium bromide in man: a study in human volunteers with special emphasis on the endocrine and the central nervous system. *Food Chem Toxicol*. 1983;21(4):409-19.

161. Sangster B et al. Study of sodium bromide in human volunteers, with special emphasis on the endocrine system. *Hum Toxicol*. 1982;1(4):393-402.

162. Vobecky M et al. Interaction of bromine with iodine in the rat thyroid gland at enhanced bromide intake. *Biol Trace Elem Res*. 1996;54(3):207-12.

163. Stasiak M et al. [Relationship between toxic effects of potassium bromate and endocrine glands]. *Endokrynol Pol*. 2009;60(1):40-50.

164. Karbownik M et al. Comparison of potential protective effects of melatonin, indole-3-proprionic acid, and propylthiouracil against lipid peroxidation caused by potassium bromate in the thyroid gland. *J Cell*

Biochem. 2005;95(1):131-8.

165. Galletti PM & Joyet G. Effect of fluorine on thyroidal iodine metabolism in hyperthyroidism. *J Clin Endocrinol Metab*. 1958;18(10):1102-1110.

166. Burgi H et al. Fluorine and thyroid gland function: a review of the literature. *Klin Wochenschr*. 1984;62(12):564-9.

167. Ristic-Medic D et al. Methods of assessment of iodine status in humans: a systematic review. *Am J Clin Nutr*. 2009;89(6(S)):2052S-69S.

168. Teng X et al. Safe range of iodine intake levels: A comparative study of thyroid diseases in three women population cohorts with slightly different iodine intake levels. *Biol Trace Elem Res*. 2007;Epub ahead of print.

169. Hurrell RF. Bioavailability of iodine. *Eur J Clin Nutr*. 1997;51(Suppl):S9-S12.

170. Gulland J. Iodine & breast health: Think beyond the thyroid. *Holistic Primary Care*. 2009;10(1):14-15.

171. Abraham GE. The bioavailability of iodine applied to the skin. *The Original Internist*. 2008;15 (2):77-79.

172. Cerqueira C et al. Association of iodine fortification with incident use of antithyroid medication - A Danish nationwide study. *J Clin Endocrinol Metab*. 2009;94(7):2400-2405.

Acknowledgements

The following practitioners have taught me extremely valuable information about how to diagnose and treat patients. Their expertise has helped me tremendously.

David M. Brady, N.D., D.C., C.C.N., D.A.C.B.N.
Jeff Moss, D.D.S., C.N.S., D.A.C.B.N.
Dietrich Klinghardt, M.D., Ph.D.
Michael Trayford, D.C., D.A.C.N.B
R. Ernest Cohn, M.D., N.M.D., D.C., F.A.C.O.
Suzannah Tebbe Davis, C.H.T., C.S.C.
David Graham, D.C.
Daniel Kalish, D.C.
Liz Lipski, Ph.D., C.C.N.
Russel Jaffe, M.D., Ph.D.
Aristo Vojdani, Ph.D.
Richard Lord, Ph.D.
Alexander Bralley, Ph.D.
Bill Kleber, D.C., D.A.B.C.I.
Frank Strehl, D.C., D.A.B.C.I.
Michael Taylor, D.C., D.A.B.C.I.
Jack Kessinger, D.C., D.A.B.C.I.
Dicken Weatherby, N.D.

About The Author

Nikolas R. Hedberg, D.C., D.A.B.C.I. treats sick patients from all over the world who have not found answers to their health problems. He is a Board Certified Internist by the American Board of Chiropractic Internists (only 200 chiropractors have achieved this designation). His Bachelor's degree is in Exercise Science from the University of Florida and his Doctor of Chiropractic is from Texas Chiropractic College. Dr. Hedberg believes that most diseases have an underlying cause that must be identified in order for a patient to truly heal.

Dr. Nik, as he is affectionately called by his patients, knew early in life that he wanted to be a doctor and help people. He was fascinated with the human body and its remarkable ability to heal. Convinced that true healing was and is possible if an individual is given the correct tools, he has brought his lifelong dream to fruition and has treated hundreds of patients with success.

Dr. Hedberg uses a variety of state-of-the-art diagnostic tests to determine the actual cause of a patient's health problem. He sees many individuals with thyroid disorders, Lyme disease, chronic fatigue syndrome, hormone imbalances and autoimmune diseases. Through his virtual practice via the Internet and telephone consultations, he is able to work with anyone regardless of location.

He is an adjunct faculty member at Hawthorn University and loves to educate patients and students about health. He has made numerous television and radio appearances and has been published in newspapers and medical journals. He also lectures throughout the United States educating doctors on alternative medicine therapies for complex conditions.

He serves as a member of the North Carolina Integrative Medical Society, The American Chiropractic Association's Council on Diagnosis & Internal Disorders, and the American Board of Chiropractic Internists. He also consults with conventional and alternative medicine physicians on complex cases.

In his spare time, Dr. Nik enjoys opera singing, skiing, meditation, yoga and hiking.